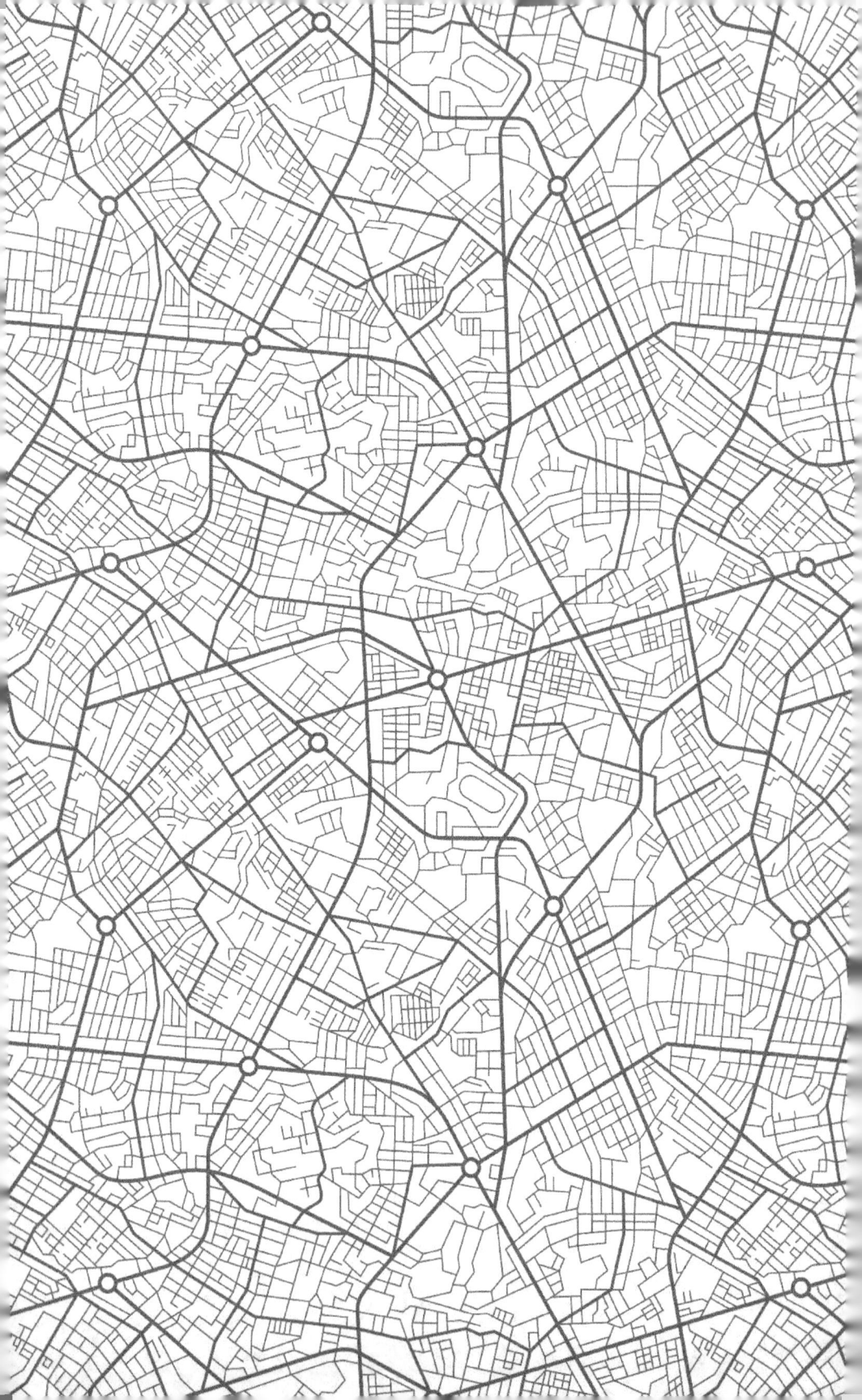

THE RHEUMATOID ARTHRITIS ROADMAP

© Donica Liu Baker 2022

For my patients,

who have taught me so much about living life to the fullest,

with or without arthritis.

Contents

Introduction — 11

Chapter 1 — 15
Navigating Your Rheumatoid Arthritis Diagnosis and Symptoms

Chapter 2 — 37
Navigating the Anti-inflammatory Diet

Chapter 3 — 59
Navigating DMARD Treatments

Chapter 4 — 115
Navigating Biologic Treatments

Chapter 5 — 149
Navigating the JAK Inhibitors

Chapter 6 — 163
Navigating Steroids and Over-the-Counter Medications

Chapter 7 — 185
Navigating Holistic, Alternative, and Complementary Approaches to Rheumatoid Arthritis

Chapter 8   **207**
Navigating Exercise, Physical Therapy,
Surgery, and Assistive Aids

Chapter 9   **221**
Navigating Rheumatoid Arthritis during
the COVID-19 Pandemic

Chapter 10   **235**
Putting It All Together

Additional Resources and   **245**
Recommended Reading

References   **247**

About the Author   **265**

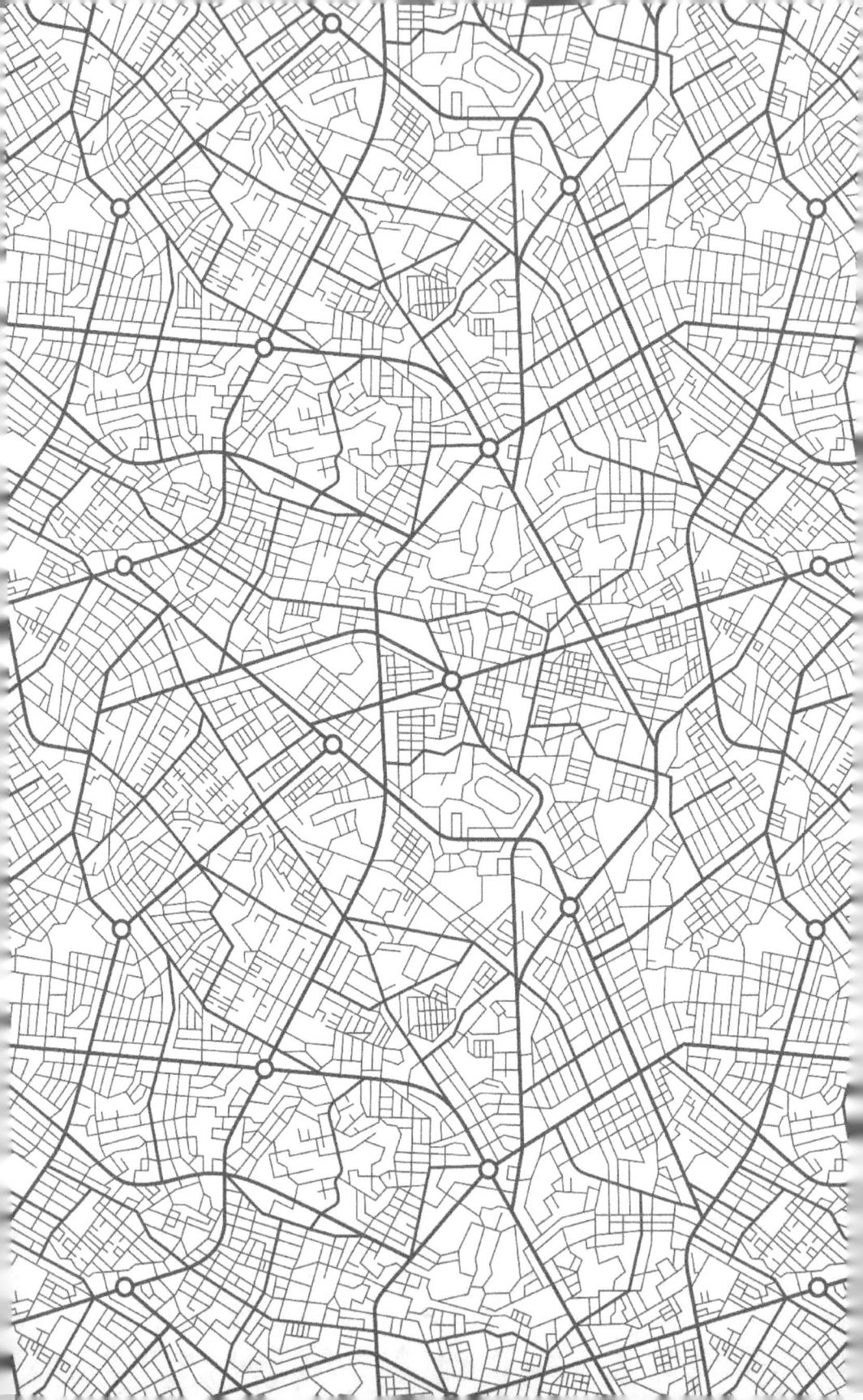

INTRODUCTION

Are you feeling lost after a new diagnosis of rheumatoid arthritis?

The experience of living with pain can be like waking up in a foreign country or a new world. Arthritis can push the pause button on your regular life and activities while you navigate through an unfamiliar place with new surroundings. Learning a new language and finding new paths to travel can be an overwhelming part of receiving a new diagnosis. Having a road map to help you navigate through this odyssey can restore some sense of control and set expectations for the journey ahead.

My patients often have mixed feelings after a recent diagnosis of rheumatoid arthritis. Which of the following points of view do you identify the most with? Write "yes" next to one or two of the following statements that apply the most to you:

- ❖ I am relieved that I finally have a diagnosis after a long search for an answer to my pain and other symptoms.
- ❖ I am devastated and disappointed that I have just been diagnosed with a chronic and painful condition that will probably require taking medications to get better.
- ❖ I'm not too surprised that I got diagnosed with rheumatoid arthritis after my joints started hurting, because it runs strongly in my family history.
- ❖ I feel neutral about my diagnosis, neither positive nor negative. I just want to be proactive about feeling better soon, whatever it takes.

❖ I'm not a medicine-taker and never have been. I would rather avoid taking medications as much as possible and take a more natural or observational approach to managing my rheumatoid arthritis.

No matter where you are or how you are feeling, please know that you're not alone and there is hope! Rheumatoid arthritis is indeed a chronic and painful condition that can affect your quality of life and mobility. The good news is that the understanding of rheumatoid arthritis is much better in the current age compared to decades ago. We have much better treatments now and most patients will not experience the degree of joint damage and deformity that occurred in the past.

Many of my patients, both young and old, are living active lives—with careers, families, hobbies, and the ability to stay fit—despite their rheumatoid arthritis. The case scenarios based on actual patients' journeys at the end of each chapter are meant to give you a window of perspective into how others are coping and living with their arthritis.

It is also up to you regarding how much treatment you want or do not want. The management of rheumatoid arthritis is a wide spectrum, ranging from mere observation and dietary changes to more intensive medical treatments. The possibilities of the anti-inflammatory diet, older and newer treatments for rheumatoid arthritis, as well as natural and holistic approaches will be discussed here.

This book has evolved with time, just as I have learned from my patients and evolved as a doctor over time. It started off as an idea to help patients understand the medications they were taking. As I saw how confused and lost patients were after being diagnosed with rheumatoid arthritis, I added information on diagnosis and symptoms, as well as navigating immunosuppression during the COVID-19 pandemic.

As I continued to listen and learn from my patients, I saw that they had a strong curiosity in the anti-inflammatory diet, supplements like turmeric, and natural approaches to reducing their inflammation. The concepts in my book grew to include an integrative philosophy and complementary approaches to rheumatoid arthritis. The result, I hope, is a contemporary, holistic, and approachable guide to rheumatoid arthritis.

I believe that transparency with patients, an honest discussion about diagnosis and potential treatments, and partnership in making shared decisions with patients is pivotal to the collaborative process that leads to successful remission of rheumatoid arthritis.

Many of my patients have shared that their new diagnosis of rheumatoid arthritis led them to recommit to self-care and living more mindfully. Although it felt like the door was closed on one area of their life, multiple other doors were opened that led to living a more intentional, fulfilling, and healthy lifestyle. I wish you the very best in your journey to health and wellness.

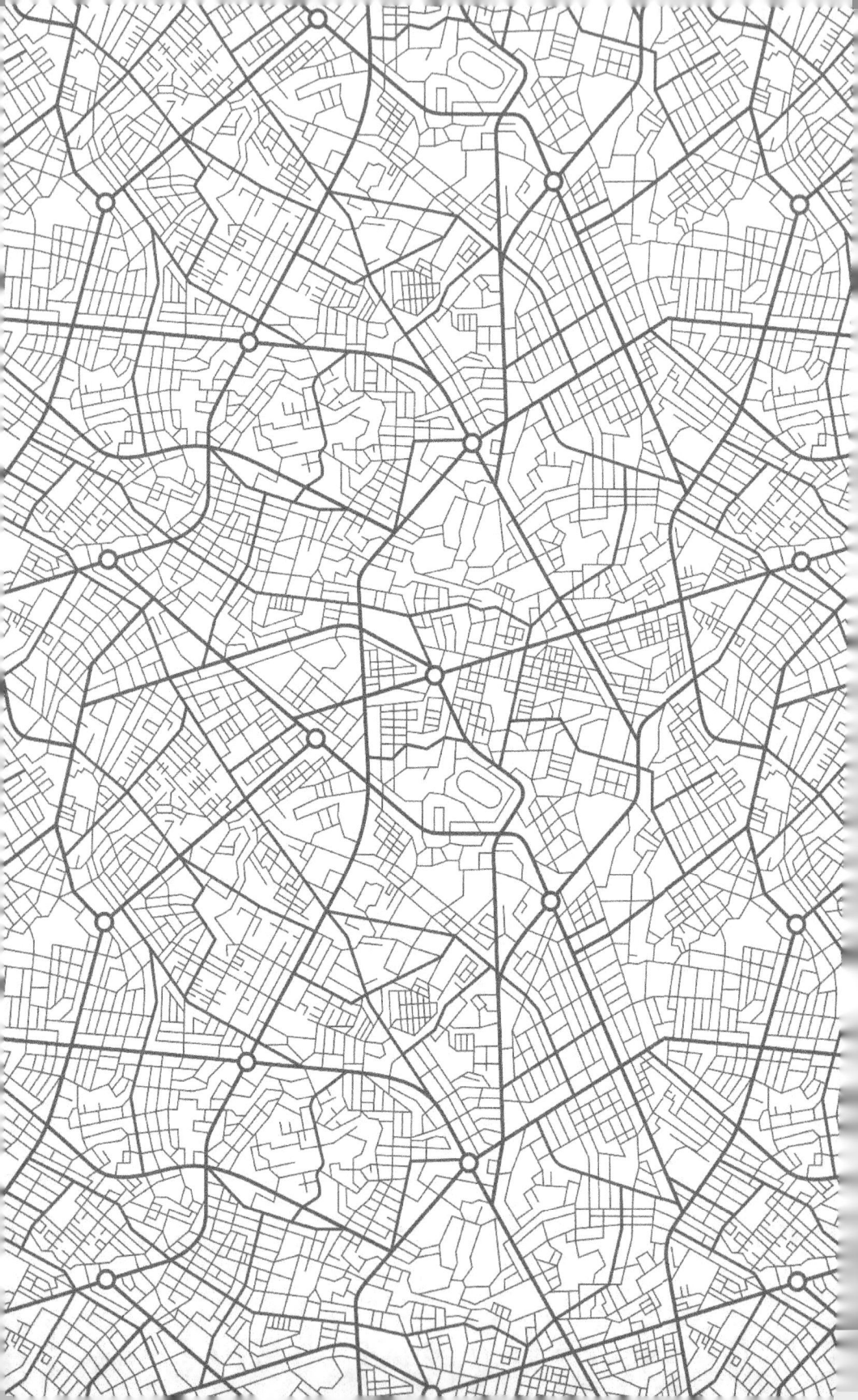

CHAPTER 1
NAVIGATING YOUR RHEUMATOID ARTHRITIS DIAGNOSIS AND SYMPTOMS

THE BASICS OF RHEUMATOID ARTHRITIS

What is rheumatoid arthritis?

Rheumatoid arthritis is a chronic autoimmune disorder that causes joint pain and swelling with increased levels of inflammation throughout the body. The synovium, which is the tissue within and around the joints, becomes inflamed and can invade into surrounding structures such as the bone, cartilage, and ligaments. Over time, this can cause joint damage and deformities to occur.

"Erosions" are the changes we see on x-rays that signify joint damage from chronic inflammation. The goal is to avoid erosions from developing.

What are autoimmune diseases?

Autoimmune diseases occur when an individual becomes the victim of his or her own immune system. Instead of attacking foreign bacteria or viruses, the immune system attacks the host's own body instead. There is a loss of "self-tolerance," when the immune system starts reacting to antigens that belong to its own body instead of recognizing them as being part of the self, and ignoring them.

How do autoimmune diseases occur?

Although still poorly understood, research has hypothesized a few mechanisms that may be involved in the development of autoimmune diseases. Typically, there is an environmental trigger in a genetically susceptible host.

The host may have been exposed to an infection or a toxin in the past that led to dysregulation of the immune system. There is also ongoing research about periodontitis (poor dental health), lung infections, or abnormal microbiology and flora of the digestive tract that can increase a person's risk of developing autoimmune disease.

What are other examples of autoimmune diseases? Could I have more than just one?

There are over eighty recognized autoimmune diseases! An autoimmune disease can be specific to one organ, such as Hashimoto thyroiditis causing hypothyroidism, or diabetes mellitus type 1 affecting the pancreas. Autoimmune diseases can also affect multiple organs or cause systemic inflammation throughout the entire body, such as rheumatoid arthritis or systemic lupus erythematosus.

Patients with one autoimmune disease can be susceptible to developing another autoimmune disease due to the dysregulation of their immune system that has occurred. For example, I have a handful of patients who have both rheumatoid arthritis as well as another autoimmune disease such as Sjogren syndrome or lupus.

Why are women affected more often by autoimmune diseases than men?

Estrogen and other hormones have been implicated in the development of autoimmune disease. Women are also more susceptible to autoimmune diseases due to their ability to bear children.

Let me explain the hypothesis of fetal microchimerism. When a baby is developing in the womb, part of his or her cells attach to the mother and enter her circulation. The fetal cells can persist in various organs in the mother up to many years after the pregnancy is over. This can lead the immune system to become confused and to lose self-tolerance.

What do the lab markers mean in rheumatoid arthritis? What is the difference between seropositive and seronegative rheumatoid arthritis?

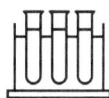

Seropositive rheumatoid arthritis is when one or both of the lab markers for rheumatoid arthritis—rheumatoid factor and anti-CCP antibodies—come back significantly positive. Typically, seropositive rheumatoid arthritis portends a more serious prognosis and can cause more rheumatoid nodules and manifestations outside the musculoskeletal system to occur.

Seronegative rheumatoid arthritis is the diagnosis when both lab markers come back negative, but there is still evidence of inflammation of the joints. For example, a rheumatologist would be able to tell if a patient has synovitis, which is swelling of the joints on the physical exam. An x-ray of the joints may also show erosions, which are the beginnings of damage from rheumatoid arthritis. Synovial fluid analysis could show an inflammatory pattern within an affected joint.

Further types of imaging such as ultrasound scans and special lab testing may rule out other types of arthritis, and reveal evidence for rheumatoid arthritis that support the diagnosis even if the two traditional lab markers are negative. There are more lab markers being studied for diagnosing rheumatoid arthritis, but they are not widely recognized or available yet at most laboratories.

Are there any newer tests that have been developed for rheumatoid arthritis that can be done in unclear cases?

The VECTRA and AVISE are newer tests that check for a panel of additional inflammatory markers in the body that are not traditionally obtained. These are tests are often utilized when patients are highly suspected to have a condition like rheumatoid arthritis, but the two traditional markers, RF and CCP, come back negative and don't correlate with the patient's symptoms.

The VECTRA test also gives a score from 0 to 100 to estimate a patient's disease activity level and can be used to predict future development of erosions on joint x-rays. It also checks blood levels of TNF and IL-6, which are inflammatory markers known to be high in patients with rheumatoid arthritis. These lab markers will be discussed in further detail in upcoming sections.

Known lab markers of rheumatoid arthritis

Rheumatoid factor (RF)
Cyclic citrullinated peptide (anti-CCP antibodies)
Anti-carbamylated protein (anti-CarP antibodies)
Protein 14-3-3
TNF alpha levels
IL-6 levels

How did I get rheumatoid arthritis?

Despite extensive research, the exact cause of rheumatoid arthritis remains largely unknown. The development of RA is thought to be multifactorial, with multiple genetic factors playing important roles. There are also environmental factors, such as tobacco smoking, silica exposure, and viral infections, which are linked to the development of RA.

How much of a role do genetics play in the development of rheumatoid arthritis?

In studies with identical twins, the concordance rate for RA was about 12 to 15%. This means that when one twin was diagnosed with RA, the other twin was diagnosed with RA about 12-15% of the time, even though they had the exact same DNA.

For fraternal twins, the concordance rate drops down to about 2-3%. This is higher than in the general population, but clearly, genetics do not confer 100% of the risk of developing RA. Many studies have estimated that genetic factors account for around 60% of an individual's susceptibility to RA.

Genetic factors related to rheumatoid arthritis

MHC region coding for HLA-DR genes
Shared epitopes found on HLA-DR4
Hypervariable regions of DNA
Polymorphisms of PTPN22 and STAT4
Epigenetic factors such as histone modification
DNA methylation

Did I get rheumatoid arthritis from a family member? Am I going to pass rheumatoid arthritis down to my children?

This is a very common question I get from patients, and I tell them that just because their mom or aunt had rheumatoid arthritis doesn't mean that they will necessarily get it too. Likewise, just because they have rheumatoid arthritis doesn't automatically mean that their children or future generations will have rheumatoid arthritis.

The risk is higher compared to the general population and for people without a family history of RA, but the correlation is not 100%.

What are environmental factors that could trigger rheumatoid arthritis?

The best recognized environmental trigger for rheumatoid arthritis is cigarette smoking. Smoking increases the odds of developing RA by twelve times. There are toxins in cigarette smoke that cause abnormal modification of proteins in the body, leading to development of anti-cyclic citrullinated proteins, otherwise known as the anti-CCP antibodies, which is one of the markers of rheumatoid arthritis.

Certain bacteria in the microflora of the mouth, lung, and gut may also contribute to development of RA. Maintaining good oral health and eating a healthy diet with lower sugar and fat content may keep your gut flora normal, which is protective against inflammation.

The "leaky gut theory" proposes that abnormalities in gastrointestinal bacteria is related to intestinal permeability and increased inflammatory response throughout the body. The leaky gut theory has also been linked to other health conditions including allergies, eczema, irritable bowel syndrome, inflammatory bowel disease, and a number of other ailments. Good nutrition to optimize gut health to decrease inflammation for rheumatoid arthritis will be discussed in an upcoming chapter.

Viruses such as the one causing infectious mononucleosis (Epstein-Barr virus) have been associated with triggering RA. Other viruses and bacteria have been identified as culprits in the development of rheumatoid arthritis as well.

Environmental triggers for rheumatoid arthritis

Cigarette smoking and tobacco use
Periodontitis from poor dental health
Abnormal digestive tract flora (leaky gut theory)
Pulmonary infections
Viral infections
Bacterial infections

Would quitting smoking help me control my rheumatoid arthritis?

Absolutely! Many of my patients have reported that quitting smoking was the single most helpful change in managing their rheumatoid arthritis and decreasing flares of pain and swelling.

One patient was even able to stop taking a lot of her medications because quitting smoking reduced so much inflammation that was in her body. Not to mention, the heart and lungs also benefit from quitting smoking, and the risk of cancer is lower.

What are the main symptoms of rheumatoid arthritis?

Rheumatoid arthritis primarily causes joint pain and swelling of the small joints of the hands and feet. Swelling can range from subtle amounts to massive swelling that is difficult to control. Although less common, rheumatoid arthritis can affect larger weight-bearing joints such as the hips or the knees.

Morning joint stiffness lasting more than an hour is also a common feature of rheumatoid arthritis. Patients also feel increased joint stiffness with being sedentary, such as sitting for long periods of time.

Patients can also develop rheumatoid nodules, which are soft and fleshy nodules that usually form over the elbows along a tendon, or over the knuckles of the fingers.

Will my joints become deformed and crooked over time?

Although this is one of the greatest concerns of both patients and rheumatologists, the joints may not necessarily become deformed over time from rheumatoid arthritis if it is caught and treated early on. If there is a lot of inflammation within the joints for long periods of time without being controlled by medications, it is a possibility that the joints could change shape over time or develop rheumatoid nodules.

Typically, with the good treatments we have these days, I rarely see a patient with deformed joints that can no longer be used. The most drastic cases I have seen are in patients who were diagnosed with rheumatoid arthritis in the 1970s or 1980s (or earlier) who didn't receive adequate treatment for many years.

Can the damage and deformities that have already occurred be reversed somehow?

Unfortunately, the damage and erosions that have already occurred in the past cannot be undone. However, the goal of treatment and management of RA is to target low disease activity level and prevent any further joint damage from occurring so that the joints can be mobile and used for as long as possible.

Can rheumatoid arthritis affect more than just my joints?

Yes, the inflammation in the body from rheumatoid arthritis can affect structures other than the joints. Notably, patients with rheumatoid arthritis have a higher risk of cardiovascular disease such as cholesterol plaques on the blood vessels of the heart due to increased inflammation within the body. It is important to maintain your health overall and reduce cardiovascular risk factors such as high blood pressure, high cholesterol, and diabetes.

Rheumatoid arthritis can affect any part of the body, but other manifestations outside the musculoskeletal system are relatively uncommon. For example, rheumatoid arthritis could affect the lining of the heart or lungs causing pericardial or pleural effusions (fluid accumulation from inflammation), but we don't see it quite as often as the joint manifestations. Rheumatoid arthritis could also cause inflammation in the eyes such as scleritis or episcleritis, or the skin causing rare type of rashes. Any organ could theoretically have more inflammation caused by rheumatoid arthritis.

Can fatigue be a significant part of rheumatoid arthritis?

Absolutely! A large portion of my rheumatoid arthritis report fatigue as a major symptom. Usually, the cause of the fatigue is multifactorial. Some of the fatigue may be due to inflammation in the body causing low energy levels. Fatigue could also be caused by joint pain at night and difficulty getting comfortable, leading to sleep disturbances.

Fatigue is one of the most difficult symptoms to treat in medicine, and is best managed with a multifaceted approach including stress reduction techniques and adding exercise as part of the treatment regimen. This can be especially difficult since arthritis patients tend to have a lot of stress and feel like they can't exercise due to joint pain. Further discussion about fatigue reduction will be included in the chapter on holistic whole health.

Can brain fog and cognitive difficulties be part of rheumatoid arthritis?

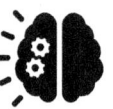

Yes, brain fog and cognitive difficulties usually go hand-in-hand with fatigue. When arthritis prevents you from sleeping well at night due to pain or other reasons, you will definitely feel brain fog, trouble processing thoughts, and word-finding difficulties, along with fatigue. A lot of patients also report that they feel like they are losing their memory and are afraid they're developing dementia or short-term memory loss.

What is the difference between rheumatoid arthritis and osteoarthritis?

Osteoarthritis is the regular wear-and-tear arthritis that everybody will get over time. Osteoarthritis starts as early as our thirties and forties, and is guaranteed to progress with age. People who do labor-intensive or physically demanding jobs, such as construction workers and professional athletes, usually develop osteoarthritis much earlier. The process of osteoarthritis is very painful and involves wearing down of cartilage and structures over time, but the immune system is not involved in attacking the body's own tissues.

On the other hand, rheumatoid arthritis involves autoimmunity and high levels of inflammation which can cause joint erosions. Whereas osteoarthritis tends to affect larger weight-bearing joints such as the hips, knees, and lower back, rheumatoid arthritis usually attacks the small joints of the hands and feet.

Is it common to have rheumatoid arthritis and osteoarthritis at the same time?

Yes, osteoarthritis is very common and we will all develop it at some point given progression of time and even with normal use of our joints and bodies. It is possible to develop an autoimmune disease such as rheumatoid arthritis in addition to having generalized osteoarthritis.

At times it can be difficult to tell which symptoms are due to osteoarthritis and which symptoms are due to rheumatoid arthritis. If you are confused, discuss your symptoms further with your rheumatologist. He or she may take more history or do more testing to distinguish between the two.

Is it possible to have rheumatoid arthritis and fibromyalgia at the same time?

Fibromyalgia is a chronic pain syndrome when people experience widespread pain, mostly in the muscles, with a sensation of invisible bruises and overactive nerves all over their body. Severe fatigue, nonrestorative sleep, and inability to exercise usually go hand-in-hand with fibromyalgia.

Patients who have experienced extreme stress, physical or emotional trauma, or high levels of pain over long periods of time are more vulnerable to developing fibromyalgia, also known as central sensitization syndrome. There is a strong association between chronic pain and *chronic cognitive-emotional hyperarousal*. This is chronic activation of the "fight or flight" responses of the sympathetic nervous system, which is a state that can lead to symptoms such as nervous system overstimulation, insomnia, anxiety, chronic headaches/migraines, irritable syndrome, and other ailments.

Unfortunately, some patients with rheumatoid arthritis have been enduring high levels of pain for so long that they do become more sensitized to pain and develop chronic pain from fibromyalgia. The best treatments for fibromyalgia are to optimize sleep, reduce stress as much as possible, practice mindfulness and meditation to reduce nervous system overstimulation, and to start a gentle form of exercise that you can do on a regular basis to rebuild strength and endurance.

Can joint paint and flares fluctuate with weather changes?

Yes, they can. It isn't just an old wives' tale that a person with arthritis can predict the weather! Barometric pressure changes in the atmosphere can induce joint pain and increased symptoms. Usually, my patients report feeling worse during cold or rainy weather. Stress and illness can also lead to flares.

Is there a cure for rheumatoid arthritis?

Currently, we don't know of a cure for autoimmune diseases such as rheumatoid arthritis. However, there are many strategies for controlling autoimmune diseases so that the condition goes "into remission," so to speak. Remission means that the condition is in low disease activity level and doesn't impact quality of life on a significant level.

Should I establish care and follow up with a rheumatologist?

It is a good idea to see a rheumatologist, a physician who is an expert on arthritis and autoimmune diseases, and follow up with him or her on a regular basis. Rheumatologists have the extensive training to diagnose you with the right type of arthritis and they are the most familiar with the type of medications used to treat rheumatoid arthritis.

Find a rheumatologist who you can communicate openly with, who is open to understanding your personal perspectives, culture, and beliefs about your health. The most healing relationship is one where communication flows openly and there is mutual trust and understanding.

Can I still live a normal life after being diagnosed with rheumatoid arthritis?

Yes. Even though things will be different than before and you may have to take new medications or change certain habits, you can still have an excellent quality of life and be an active person. A lot of my patients with rheumatoid arthritis feel that they are living a relatively normal and healthy life.

A small percentage of patients have a really severe and aggressive form of rheumatoid arthritis, and they experience frequent flares with weather changes or increased stress. Some of these patients are taking a more intensive medication regimen than others and they miss a couple weeks of work every year due to their flares. I don't think everyone would describe their life as "normal" with rheumatoid arthritis, but overall, most people feel their condition is manageable at baseline with occasional flares.

Will I be able to continue working and taking care of my family with rheumatoid arthritis?

Yes. It may initially take some time to get your rheumatoid arthritis under control. Medications usually take around 2-3 months to build up to therapeutic levels in your body. During this time, it can feel like you're stuck in purgatory, just waiting for the day when you start to feel better. Eventually, your joints and symptoms will start to improve.

You will reach a new baseline level of functioning. For some, this may be returning to how they felt in the past, or mostly living pain-free and with occasional flares once or twice per year that cause minimal interference with their life. For others, this may mean living with more pain on a day-to-day basis that is tolerable and controllable, but not quite the same as they felt before.

You may be someone who was really independent, always taking care of others, and a hard worker who is always doing things for everyone else. For a little while, you may be in a period of life where other people are taking care of you and helping you out until you can get back on your feet and adjusted to a new health condition. We all have seasons of life where we have to lean more on others, and it's okay to depend on others for help. It's okay to ask your family and friends for more assistance and understanding during this time.

Will I become disabled eventually?

Not necessarily. Permanent disability from rheumatoid arthritis is considered rare in the current era. There is a small percentage of patients with severe rheumatoid arthritis who do end up experiencing destruction of their joints and have to leave their job and assume fewer responsibilities within their family. I would say this is few and far between compared to the other cases of successful recovery.

Most of my younger patients are working and living productive lives. Some of my patients are older and retired, but they still participate in gardening, fishing, and other activities.

Case scenarios

These case scenarios are illustrations of journeys that different patients may experience, which are loosely based on the paths that some of my patients have taken to arrive at their diagnosis. Names have been changed for anonymity.

Case 1

Cathy is a dental hygienist who has always loved her work. Recently she has had more trouble working with the dental tools and has noticed decreased grip strength and manual dexterity of her hands. She has experienced joint pain and swelling, as well as more fatigue, in the past year or so.

She sought evaluation from her primary care doctor and was referred to a rheumatologist. She was found to have high levels of both the rheumatoid factor and anti-CCP antibodies on her bloodwork. Hand x-rays showed the early beginnings of erosions on her hand joints.

Cathy and her rheumatologist discussed her new diagnosis of severe seropositive rheumatoid arthritis. Cathy was confused about how she even got rheumatoid arthritis in the first place. The diagnosis seemed really out of the blue since nobody in her family ever had arthritis and she never did anything to make herself unhealthy.

As a busy working mom of three children, she was worried about maintaining her job and family life, both of which required heavy use of her hands. She and her rheumatologist discussed starting treatments early on as an aggressive strategy to prevent further damage to her joints.

Case 2

John was always very fit and active, ran marathons every year and worked a busy job in sales. Recently he has felt like a "90-year-old man trapped inside a 42-year-old's body." At this young age, he started experiencing joint pain and swelling in his hands and feet, as well as an aching sensation throughout his entire body.

At first, he thought he was just overdoing things and took a break from running marathons and cut back on extra work hours. Even with scaling back on his activity level, his joint pain got worse and he started having trouble keeping up with his two kids. He took a lot of ibuprofen and Tylenol every day just to get through the day. His family practice doctor also gave him a prednisone taper to see if it would help him, and it did, but only for a temporary period of time.

After seeing a rheumatologist for joint pain, he tested negative for rheumatoid factor but positive for the anti-CCP antibodies, and was diagnosed with seropositive rheumatoid arthritis. His x-rays turned out to be normal. John was never a medicine taker, and was hesitant to take any long-term medications, but he discussed potential therapies with his rheumatologist to see which one would be the best fit for him. He didn't want to be on medications for the rest of his life, but he also didn't want to live with chronic joint pain and decreased mobility, so he decided to go ahead and start one of the first-line medications.

Case 3

Anna started experiencing joint pain as a young child at the age of three. Her mom noticed that she was having trouble walking and her knees and ankles were looking red and swollen. She was diagnosed with juvenile arthritis by a pediatric rheumatologist. As Anna entered adolescence, her arthritis symptoms seemed to go into remission, and she was able to get through high school and college with no major setbacks.

However, when Anna started nursing school after college, she experienced return of joint pain and swelling in her knees and ankles. She started having trouble attending classes and nursing clinicals due to trouble walking and standing for long periods of time that is required of nurses.

Anna established care with an adult rheumatologist and had large quantities of fluid drawn out from her swollen knee joints. The synovial fluid analysis showed high levels of inflammation even though the rheumatoid factor and anti-CCP antibodies came back normal several times on her blood work. A VECTRA blood test showed that she had a high score correlating with a high probability of having rheumatoid arthritis.

She and her rheumatologist felt that the arthritis she had when she was younger became active again in adulthood, and she was diagnosed with seronegative rheumatoid arthritis. They discussed potential treatments together so that she could reach her full potential in school and become the nurse she was meant to be.

Action list:

- ☐ Start a log or diary of all of your symptoms and possible links with triggers such as stress or weather changes that lead to flares.
- ☐ Write down any initial thoughts and fears about your new diagnosis. See reflection questions on the next page if you need guidance.
- ☐ Find out whether your labs show if you have seropositive or seronegative rheumatoid arthritis.
- ☐ Find out whether your baseline x-rays show any joint damage starting to occur.
- ☐ Talk to family members and relatives, and find out whether you have any history of arthritis or autoimmune diseases in your family tree.
- ☐ Make a list of other questions or concerns you have for your rheumatologist.

Reflection questions:

1. What are your greatest fears about rheumatoid arthritis after diagnosis?

2. What are the most challenging symptoms you have been coping with so far?

3. What have been the biggest changes in your life after diagnosis?

4. What still confuses you about your rheumatoid arthritis diagnosis or symptoms?

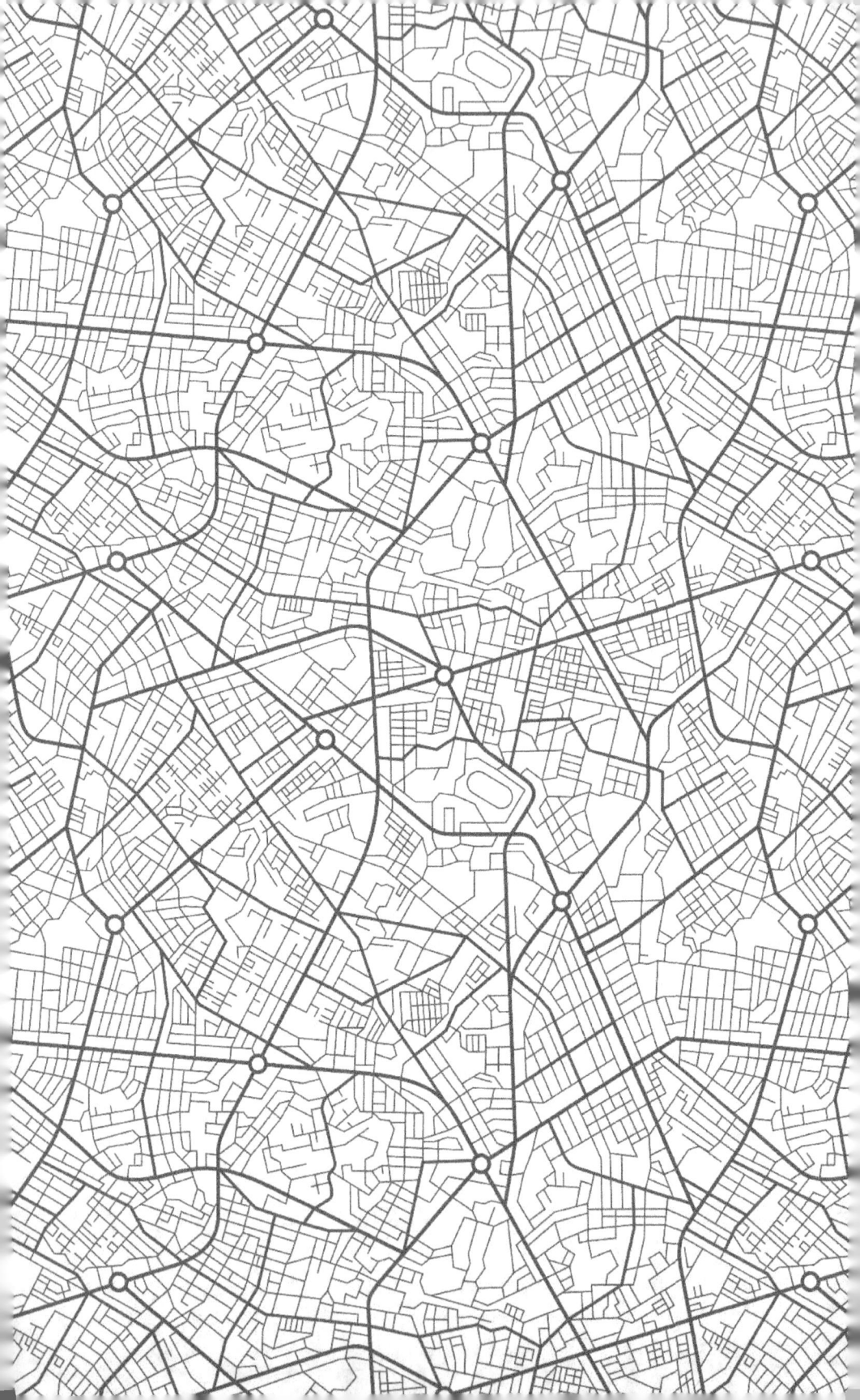

CHAPTER 2
NAVIGATING THE ANTI-INFLAMMATORY DIET

THE ANTI-INFLAMMATORY DIET IN A NUTSHELL

"Eat food. Not too much. Mostly plants."
[Michael Pollan]

What is an "anti-inflammatory diet"?

Although it may sound mysterious, an anti-inflammatory diet is just eating healthy in general! This means eating more fruits and vegetables, and less animal products like meat. Red meats, especially, produce more inflammation in the body. Reducing red meat intake such as steak or hamburger is an important part of the anti-inflammatory diet.

Adding spices like turmeric and ginger to your food, if you don't mind the taste of these spices, can also be helpful. If you're able to, cook most of your food from scratch at home using fresh ingredients, rather than eating out at restaurants or heating pre-packaged meals.

The most anti-inflammatory diet is a completely plant-based and vegan diet, but this may be difficult to abide by, and it may be challenging to find good sources of protein and essential micronutrients such as vitamin B12 which is only found in animal products. Moderation is usually easier to achieve and more realistic to maintain than drastic and sudden changes in your eating habits.

Can eating a healthy diet help control my rheumatoid arthritis symptoms?

Overall, eating a healthy diet will help every part of your body! Not only will your arthritis get better, but your high cholesterol and high blood pressure would also improve if you have those conditions too. The anti-inflammatory diet is very similar to the Mediterranean diet for heart health and diabetes. The Mediterranean diet encourages increased fruits and vegetables, extra virgin olive oil, fish rich in omega-3 fatty acids, and intake of nuts such as almonds, walnuts, and pecans.

The Okinawan diet is another model of the anti-inflammatory diet. The Okinawa prefecture is on a small tropical island off the southern coast of Japan. Residents of Okinawa are known for their long life expectancy and low use of medications. They have the highest number of centenarians (citizens who live to age 100 and above) and have a low rate of age-associated diseases such as obesity, diabetes, high blood pressure, and arthritis.

Healthcare spending is overall low in Japan but the healthcare outcomes are very positive compared to other countries. The Okinawans eat a diet that is low in calories but full of nutrients and antioxidants. I also follow the Okinawan saying that "you should eat until you're about 80% full and then stop." This helps you listen to your body's signals to stop filling up, and prevents overeating.

Cutting out unhealthy foods will decrease the levels of inflammation in your body and help you on your way to living with less pain. The joints are also very sensitive to excess weight, so shedding a few pounds if you are overweight would decrease the biomechanical load that your joints have to carry. Here are some basic principles of the anti-inflammatory diet.

Eat more:

- **Colorful whole fruits and vegetables**—foods with deep red, yellow, orange, and green colors that contain

antioxidants, vitamins, and minerals. Berries are strong antioxidants!
- **Healthy fats**—including omega-3 fatty acids from fish such as salmon, mackerel, and sardines, and foods such as avocados, extra virgin olive oil, raw nuts, and seeds.
- **Fiber**—creates a favorable environment for healthy bacteria in your gut, promotes adequate bowel movements which makes your gut happy, and supports the body's detoxification process. Adding a few tablespoons of ground flaxseeds daily is a great way to add fiber to your diet.
- **Organic grass-fed beef or bison**—higher in anti-inflammatory essential fats such as omega-3 fatty acids. Grass-fed beef also contains fewer calories and less bacteria. Organic free-range chicken is lower in antibiotics which is a cleaner source of protein.
- **Spices and herbs**—seasonings such as garlic, ginger, and turmeric add a flavorful anti-inflammatory component to the diet.

Eat less:

- **Trans or hydrogenated fats**—the body has no mechanism to process and breakdown these unnatural fats that ultimately build up in your body and cause inflammation. Reduce these unhealthy fats as much as possible.
- **Refined oils**—commercial safflower, corn, and canola oils can be converted to arachidonic acid, which is a type of fat that stimulates higher inflammation in the body. Avoid fried foods which are soaked in these unhealthy oils.

- **High glycemic foods**—refined carbohydrates such as breads, pastas, cakes, candy (all the "good stuff"), fruit juice, and corn syrup leads to a rapid rise in blood sugar and an inflammatory cascade stimulated by insulin.
- **Processed or packaged foods**—avoid the frozen aisle of the grocery store! Avoid canned foods and eat fresh foods instead. Unprocess your food as much as possible and cook from scratch instead.
- **Red meats**—such as steak and hamburgers. If you are really craving a burger once in a while, eat one that is made from grass-fed beef instead!
- **Artificial sweeteners and preservatives**—these have no nutritional value and promote inflammation. Avoid artificial colors, flavors, dyes, and other artificial ingredients. Reduce the consumption of sodas and sugary drinks.

Should I eat gluten free?

The gluten-free diet can be a bit controversial. If you have Celiac disease, it's pretty clear-cut that you should avoid gluten and gluten cross-contamination. There are also people who are known to have "non-celiac gluten sensitivity" who don't have the blood markers for Celiac disease, but definitely have symptoms when they consume gluten. If you don't have a formal diagnosis of Celiac disease, but know for sure that eating gluten products makes you feel bad based on experimentation, then it's advisable to avoid it as well.

Overall, eating a lot of wheat and carbohydrates from bread and pasta is considered "inflammatory." By reducing these carbs from the diet, patients say that they generally feel better, lose weight, and have less joint pain. For most people who don't have Celiac disease or the "non-celiac gluten sensitivity," there's no strict guidelines on whether to avoid gluten completely or not.

You could experiment with reducing or eliminating gluten from your diet to see how it makes you feel. You could also choose to keep some gluten in your diet, but just eat it in moderation without overdoing it.

Should I reduce my consumption of sugar?

I have some patients who swear by reducing sugar from their diet to control their rheumatoid arthritis. If they eat too much cake or ice cream, "they feel it in their joints."

Again, there's no strict guidelines regarding sugar, but moderating sugar in your diet is a good plan overall. A high blood glucose is known to increase inflammation in the body, not to mention it increases the risk of diabetes mellitus and obesity as well. An exception to reducing sugar is dark chocolate. Dark chocolate contains high levels of flavonoids and antioxidants, and serves as an occasional treat. Good news for chocolate lovers!

Should I avoid dairy products?

When patients ask what my personal opinion of dairy products is and whether I eat them or not, I tell them that I am unfortunately lactose intolerant and can't eat a lot of dairy to begin with. To find out whether your body is sensitive to dairy or not, eliminate it from your diet for 2 weeks or more and see how you feel. If you feel much better, you could leave dairy out long-term. If there's no difference in how you feel, you could add dairy back in. Take this elimination approach with any ingredient or suspected food allergen to see if it makes a difference in how you feel.

The Leaky Gut Theory

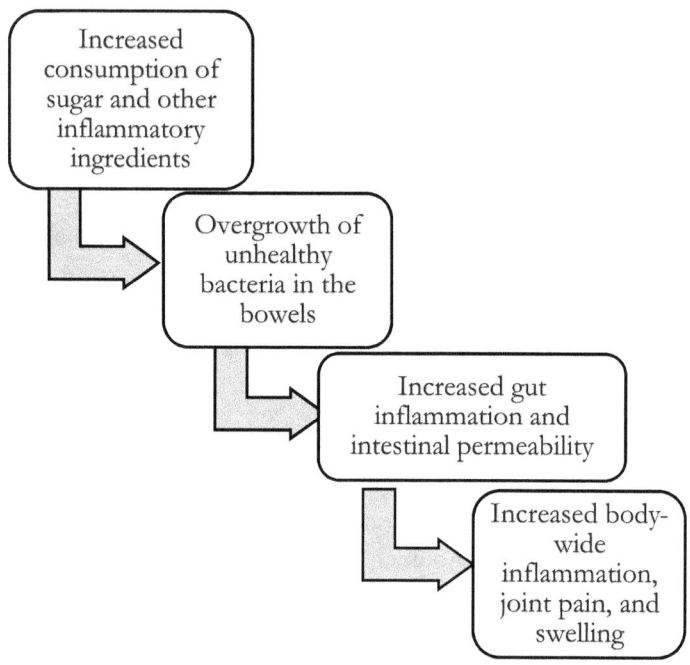

Steps in the Elimination Diet

Step 1	**Planning phase:** identify food culprits that you suspect may be playing a role in your symptoms. For example, gluten, dairy, sugar, preservatives, artificial dyes, red meats, etc.
Step 2	**Avoidance phase:** eliminate one food or an entire food group for at least 2 to 4 weeks. Note that symptoms may worsen before they start to improve.

Step 3	**Challenge phase:** reintroduce culprit food or ingredient back into diet to see if it exacerbates symptoms.
Step 4	Create a long-term diet plan based on results. Repeat steps for other suspected food culprits.

Should I start taking turmeric supplements?

Of course, no discussion about defying inflammation would be complete without including turmeric, the golden queen of anti-inflammatory spices! Turmeric is a spice commonly used in Indian and Middle Eastern cuisine. Turmeric is often added in curry dishes and has a bright yellow appearance. It typically comes in a powder derived from the turmeric root, which looks like ginger or ginseng.

A lot of my patients are taking turmeric supplements to fight inflammation, which can help. Turmeric isn't going to cure arthritis on its own, but it can be part of healthful eating. It is better to get turmeric in its natural form and sprinkle some in your food every now and then, if you don't mind the taste, rather than taking it in a capsule or pill form. A tip is that eating some black pepper with turmeric increases its potency!

Would turmeric have any interactions with any of the medications I am taking?

Turmeric has some drug interactions with medications that are blood thinners. It can increase the effects of blood thinners like warfarin, but you would have to eat a whole lot of it to make a significant difference.

Overall, a little sprinkle of turmeric in your food or around 1000 mg of it as a supplement is considered harmless.

Mechanism of Action

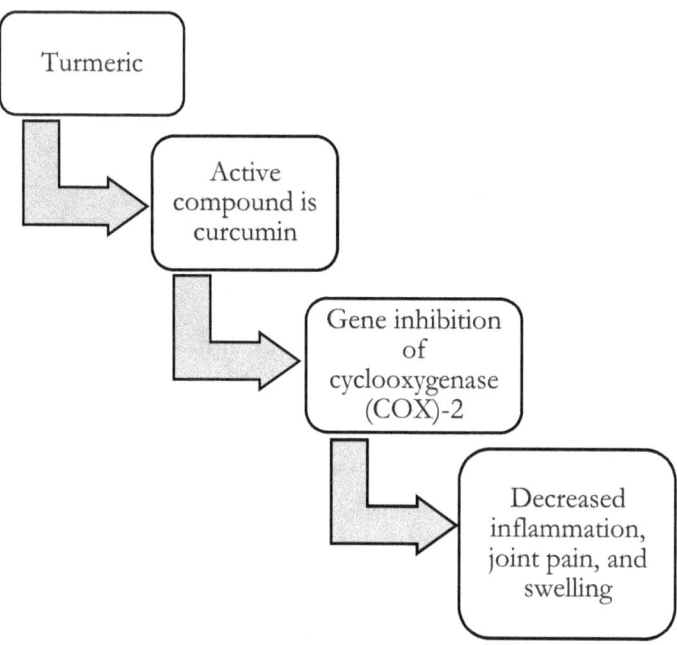

What is an easy way to get started with the anti-inflammatory diet?

An easy way to get started with the anti-inflammatory diet is to replace one or two things you commonly eat with ingredients that fight inflammation. For example, instead of baking with regular wheat flour and white refined sugar, you could replace those ingredients with almond flour and coconut sugar.

Instead of eating regular pasta all the time, try zucchini noodles (lovingly called "zoodles" by fans) once in a while. If you enjoy bubbly sodas, change your drinks to carbonated flavored water instead, which still has flavor but no sugar or artificial ingredients.

Over time, healthy ingredients and habits build up more and more while unhelpful ingredients start becoming eliminated. This is a gradual approach to eating healthier without having to do a drastic overhaul of your entire fridge and pantry all at once.

Remember that eating healthy doesn't necessarily have to be complicated. In fact, the healthiest foods are ones taken straight from the earth without any preparation done to them or ingredients added to them. Take an organic cucumber or tomato from the earth, and don't add any salt, sugar, or oil to it. Don't fry it, grill it, barbecue, or bake it. Just eat the natural foods that the earth has to offer to you, enjoy their natural flavors, and that will be plenty anti-inflammatory!

Have you ever noticed that eating healthier can actually save time and money? I used to hate it when I forgot to defrost meat ahead of time and dinner was delayed because the meat wasn't ready. Buying steak and other meats were always the more expensive items on my shopping list. Now I'm mostly buying vegetables from Aldi's to make a different veggie stir fry every night for dinner with a healthy oil. It has saved so much time and money. In fact, once in a while when I'm feeling "lazy" about meal preparation, I will just eat some raw fruits and vegetables and call it a cleansing day—both refreshing and requires minimal effort!

Live an anti-inflammatory lifestyle! Reduce stress as much as possible, get enough sleep, exercise on a regular basis if you can, prioritize self-care, and practice gratitude, patience, and forgiveness towards others. Stay positive, laugh every day, sing in the shower, dance in your kitchen, and have fun with your loved ones.

When you wake up every morning, say to yourself, "I'm going to stay positive today, no matter what comes my way and regardless of what other people say or do." Keep weight under control, eat mindfully, and spice it up!

Instead of...	Try this instead...
Regular baking flour	Almond flour
White sugar	Brown sugar or coconut sugar
Regular wheat pasta	Zucchini noodles (zoodles), palm heart noodles, or rice noodles
Regular ground beef	Grass fed ground beef or bison
Regular or diet soda	LaCroix sparkling water, San Pellegrino (or another brand)
Corn oil	Avocado oil Extra virgin olive oil
Dairy milk	Almond milk or oat milk
Canned vegetables and fruits	Fresh vegetables and fruits
Splenda or artificial sweeteners	Honey
Eating out at restaurants too often	Meal prep kits at home such as "Hello Fresh" or "Home Chef"
Coffee with cream and sugar	Chai tea which contains ginger and anti-inflammatory spices, or green tea which is full of antioxidants

Mechanism of Action

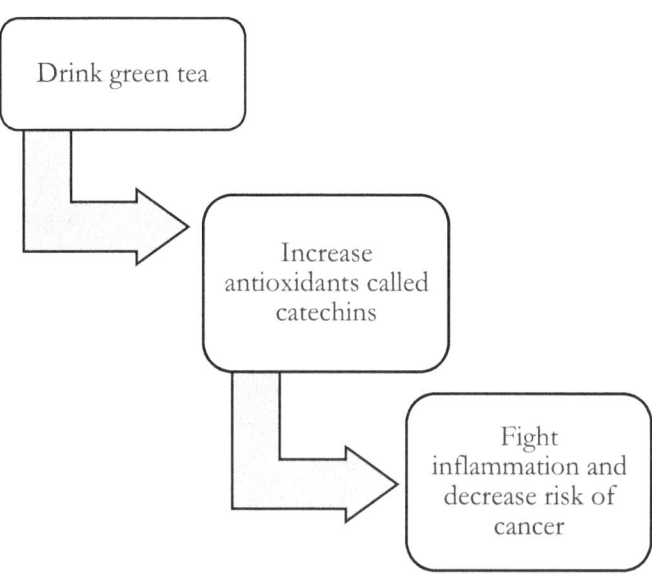

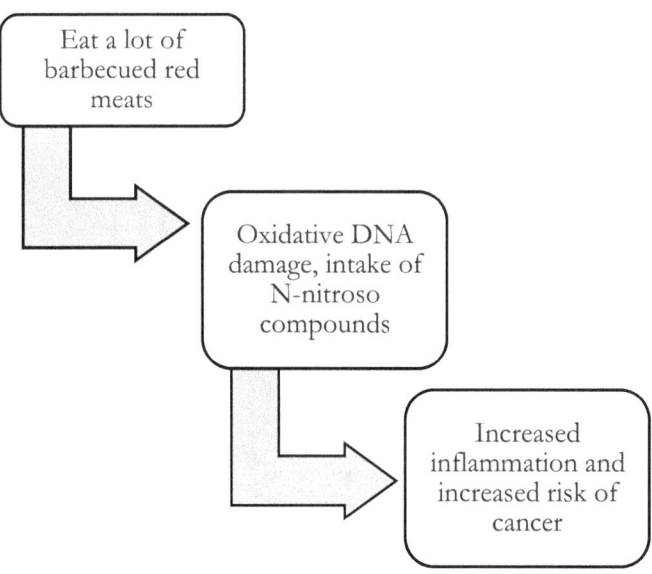

Where can I find some anti-inflammatory recipes?

There are many anti-inflammatory cookbooks sold online and in bookstores. There are also many websites devoted to recipes that fight inflammation. A book I have recommended to a lot of my patients is the "The Complete Anti-inflammatory Diet for Beginners" by Dorothy Calimeris and Lulu Cook, available at any bookstore and online.

On the following pages, there are some recipes straight from my own kitchen for you to try! These recipes are free of gluten, dairy, artificial ingredients, and refined sugars. A tip for cooking with arthritis—if cutting vegetables hurts your hand and wrist joints too much, buy precut veggies from the grocery store instead!

Golden Turmeric Curry

This recipe has a light curry flavor, and is full of spices like turmeric and ginger to help fight inflammation.

Vegetables:

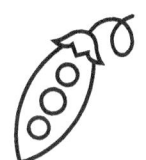

- 4 stalks of celery
- 1 fennel heart (remove stems)
- 3 medium carrots, peeled
- 1 small package of sugar snap peas

Spices:

- 1/2 teaspoon ginger fresh or powdered
- 1/4 teaspoon turmeric powder
- 1/2 teaspoon curry powder, add more if you'd like
- 1/8 teaspoon cloves
- 1/8 teaspoon cinnamon
- 1/2 teaspoon fennel seed
- 1 star anise (optional)
- 1 tablespoon apple cider vinegar
- Salt and pepper to taste

Directions:
Let's keep this simple. Cut all vegetables into bite-sized pieces. Heat avocado oil in pan and stir fry vegetables for 2 minutes until light brown. Add 1 cup of vegetable or chicken broth, cover, and simmer for 3 minutes. Add spices, salt, and pepper to taste. Simmer until vegetables are softened to your liking, about 5 minutes total.

Serve with white or brown jasmine rice.

Chilean Sea Bass

Tired of salmon and tilapia? Try some wild-caught Chilean sea bass to get your omega-3 fatty acids instead!

Ingredients:

- One small to medium piece of Chilean sea bass
- 1 tablespoon olive oil or avocado oil
- 1/2 cup chicken or vegetable broth
- 1/2 cup white cooking wine
- 1/3 cup soy sauce
- 1 teaspoon apple cider vinegar

Directions:

Heat oil in pan on medium heat. Place sea bass in pan when oil hasn't gotten extremely hot. As oil starts to sizzle, pour in broth, cooking wine, vinegar, and soy sauce.

Cover and allow to gently simmer for 5 minutes. Remove from heat and garnish with parsley and green onions if you'd like.

Serve with white or brown jasmine rice. As a side dish, you could serve green beans or another vegetable.

Favorite Veggie Stir Fry

Ingredients:

- Baby bok choy
- 1 small or medium package of soybean sprouts
- Bamboo shoots, either whole or pre-sliced
- Shiitake mushrooms
- Diced white onions
- 2 tablespoons miso paste
- 1 teaspoon apple cider vinegar
- 1 tablespoon grapeseed oil
- 1/2 teaspoon ginger fresh or powdered
- 1 teaspoon soy sauce (can substitute with gluten free soy sauce)
- Salt and pepper to taste
- 1/3 cup vegetable broth

Directions:

Heat grapeseed oil in pan and add white onions. After onions are lightly browned, add chopped baby bok choy, bamboo shoots, mushrooms, and the soybean sprouts. Stir fry for 1-2 minutes, then pour in the vegetable broth.

Add the miso paste and let it dissolve. Add the vinegar, ginger, salt, and pepper. Let simmer uncovered until the baby bok choy has a vibrant green color, about 5 minutes.

Homemade Chai Tea Latte

Loaded with anti-inflammatory spices like ginger, this recipe is simple and I keep a jug full of pre-made tea in my fridge to drink every day. So much better than Starbucks!

Ingredients:

- 6 black tea bags, any type or brand
- 1 piece freshly sliced ginger, about 2 inches
- 2 cinnamon sticks
- 2 teaspoons whole black peppercorn
- 10 whole cloves
- 6 green cardamom pods, cracked
- 4 cups of water
- Almond or oat milk
- Local honey

Directions:

Bring water to boil in medium pot. Add ginger and spices. Simmer for 5-7 minutes. Remove from heat and steep the tea bags in the liquid for 10 minutes. Strain the tea using a mesh into a pitcher or teapot, or remove all solid ingredients using a slotted spoon.

When ready to serve, add honey if you would like to sweeten. Fill half of your cup or mug with tea mixture and the other half with milk of your choice.

Case scenarios

These case scenarios are illustrations of journeys that different patients may experience, which are loosely based on the paths that some of my patients have taken with the anti-inflammatory diet. Names have been changed for anonymity.

Case 1

Lisa, a patient with seropositive rheumatoid arthritis, doesn't take any medications for her arthritis, and controls it mostly by eating a very strict anti-inflammatory diet. The effort she has put into modifying her diet and has changed her entire lifestyle, but she feels it is worth it to feel better while taking less medications.

Lisa has eliminated all gluten, dairy, and sugar from her diet. If she bakes, she uses almond flour, and she drinks almond milk or oat milk instead of dairy milk. For her birthday, she had a "cheat day" and ate a lot of cake and ice cream with her friends. The next day, she felt a flare of her rheumatoid arthritis with increased joint pain, swelling, and fatigue for about a week until she recovered.

Case 2

Vicki was sick and tired of taking so many medications for her rheumatoid arthritis. She felt like she took handful of pills every morning and wanted to remove as many unnecessary prescription medications from her list as possible. She read online that she could feel better by natural methods like drinking green smoothies and taking turmeric.

Vicki stopped all of her rheumatoid arthritis medications to see how she would feel. She made a tremendous effort at the anti-inflammatory diet, and changing aspects of her lifestyle to get healthier. After 6 months, she had made great progress and even lost some weight, but she still experienced frequent flares of her rheumatoid arthritis symptoms. She decided to go back on one or two of her medications to feel better, while continuing the diet and lifestyle changes she had started.

Case 3

Robert hasn't had any issues or side effects from taking his rheumatoid arthritis medications, so he continues to take them regularly as prescribed. In addition to medications, he read about some vitamins and supplements he could add to his regimen to reduce inflammation. He added a turmeric capsule and a fish oil supplement to his list and feels that they have been helpful.

Action list:

- ☐ Start with one or two healthy replacements for inflammatory ingredients in your food.

- ☐ Find an anti-inflammatory cookbook that looks interesting to you and try out one of the recipes (or look up a free recipe online to try).

- ☐ Get a small jar of turmeric from the grocery store and see if you could try a small sprinkle of it in the meals you're eating this week.

- ❐ Make a list of any other questions you have for your rheumatologist about the anti-inflammatory diet.

- ❐ Try an elimination diet for any food ingredients that you have suspected to be a trigger.

Reflection questions:

1. What foods are you eating that could be increasing inflammation in your body?

2. Do you feel more joint pain and fatigue after eating certain foods?

3. What aspects of the anti-inflammatory diet seem like the most challenging hurdles to overcome?

4. What is an "inflammatory" ingredient that you regularly include in your diet that you could eliminate and replace with an "anti-inflammatory" ingredient?

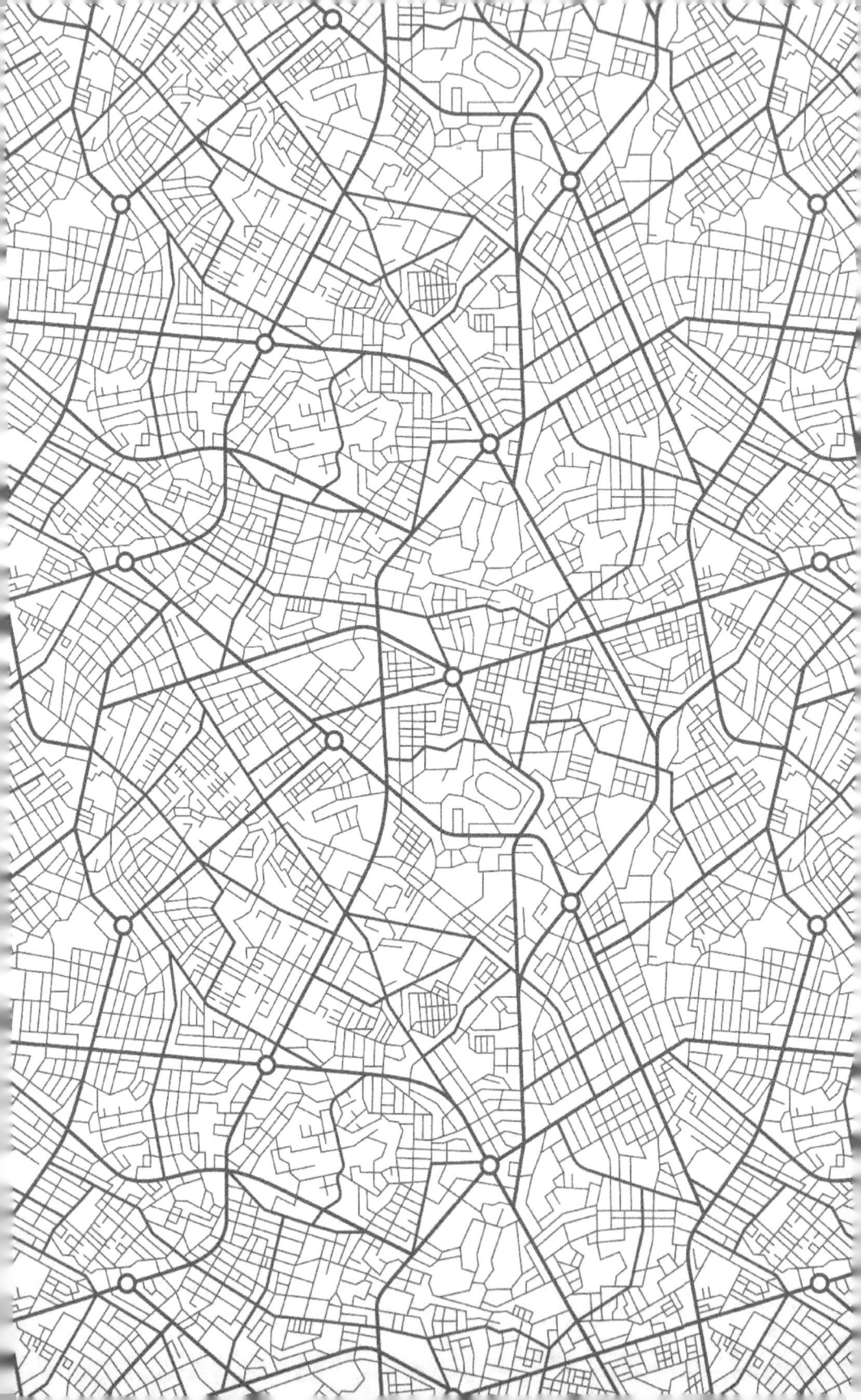

CHAPTER 3

NAVIGATING DMARD TREATMENTS

FIRST-LINE THERAPIES FOR RHEUMATOID ARTHRITIS

What are older medications for rheumatoid arthritis that were used as the initial treatments?

Before rheumatoid arthritis was established as a well-known condition, and before we had proven treatments for RA, patients were living with horrendous joint pain without real answers or solutions. They were taking handfuls of ibuprofen just to get by in their daily lives. They would develop kidney injury and gastrointestinal bleeding due to large doses of ibuprofen, but they had no other choice for controlling their joint pain.

In the 1980s, patients started receiving gold injections for treatment of their RA. I still have some older patients who recall this experience and tell me stories about when they were on gold injections. Gold compounds were meant to block certain inflammatory substances in the body, but are no longer made or used for rheumatoid arthritis.

Eventually, with better understanding of the inflammatory nature of RA, more research was available on how to treat this condition and prevent crippling of the hands and other joints over time. Very rarely do we see patients nowadays with bent and deformed fingers, unless the patient's diagnosis wasn't caught or treated early on. With early detection and treatment of RA, joint damage can be entirely avoided.

What is the first line treatment for rheumatoid arthritis in the current age?

Since the discovery of DMARD medications around the 1950s to 1980s, they have been increasingly used for rheumatoid arthritis and other types of autoimmune diseases such as psoriatic arthritis and lupus. Nowadays, DMARD medications such as methotrexate are used as first-line treatments for rheumatoid arthritis.

Most patients diagnosed with rheumatoid arthritis will have tried methotrexate at least once in their lives unless they have a contraindication such as liver disease. There are a few medications within the DMARD family which will be discussed both as a group and also individually below.

What are potential benefits of taking one of the older medications over one of the newer treatments?

Since DMARDs have been around for a while, we know much more about them and how to monitor for side effects compared to the newer biologic therapies. They have a proven efficacy and long-lasting protection for the joints.

DMARDs also come as tablets which is convenient to take for patients who want to avoid injections and needles.

What are important aspects of treatment to consider before starting any medication?

1. **Is the medication meant for symptom suppression or symptom resolution?** We will discuss whether treatments for rheumatoid arthritis are just covering up the symptoms or actually addressing the underlying issues of inflammation and autoimmune disease. We will go over whether certain medications have long-term protective effects for the joints or whether they are a temporary fix.

2. **What is the evidence for using this medication?** We will discuss whether research has proven a benefit from taking these medications and how they actually work in the body.

3. **What are the potential harms of taking this medication?** Any medication could come with side effects, which have to be considered and monitored over time. The risks and benefits have to be weighed to see whether it's worth it to take the medication.

4. **Does this therapy match my personal culture and beliefs about health?** Everyone has a different preference for treatment based on how they grew up, the people around them, and their previous experiences with healthcare. Ideally, taking a medication should fit your personal and cultural preferences.

5. **What is the cost?** Medications should be affordable to patients and accessible to those who need them. We will be reviewing the financial and insurance aspects of different treatments.

What is an integrative approach to managing rheumatoid arthritis?

An integrative approach is taking the entire body and "whole health" into account, rather than treating each body part as a separate disconnected entity. Integrative medicine honors the intricate connection between, mind, body, and spirit, and stays open-minded towards natural and holistic approaches to managing chronic pain and fatigue.

Instead of just focusing on prescription medications and invasive procedures like joint surgery, this approach takes multiple viewpoints in the spectrum of heath maintenance into consideration, and works collaboratively with other disciplines such as chiropractics, Eastern medicine, or complementary treatments. Lifestyle interventions such as nutrition, dietary changes, exercise, and stress reduction are also important pieces of integrative medicine.

The benefit of integrative medicine is that it can more closely match a patient's individual beliefs, culture, and preferences about his or her own health. It can also help with minimizing expensive healthcare costs and delay the need for more invasive measures such as surgery. The challenge or drawback of this approach is making sure that holistic therapies are evidence-based and safe for patients. Looking at research studies and strength of recommendations can help prevent both patients and doctors from buying into fraudulent claims.

While prescription medications are extensively researched and stringently regulated by the FDA, there are no quality or safety measures in place to monitor alternative therapies, which can result in unclear benefits and side effects of these treatments. This means that doctors and patients usually have to do more of their own research in understanding these treatments.

The Integrative Approach to Arthritis

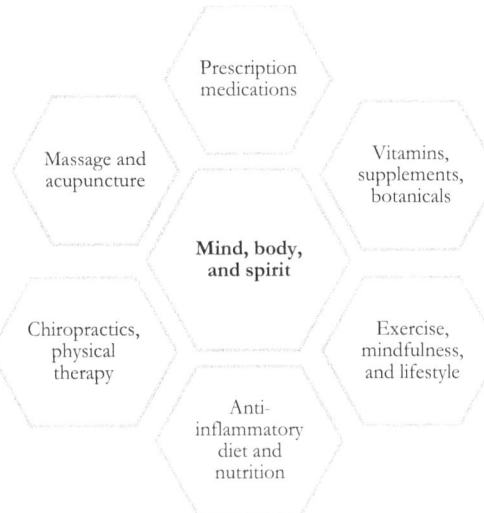

DISEASE-MODIFYING ANTI-RHEUMATIC DRUGS

"Everything is a risk. Not doing anything is a risk. It's up you."
[from the book Everything, Everything by Nicola Yoon]

What are DMARDs?

The term "DMARD" stands for disease-modifying anti-rheumatic drug." Since this is a mouthful, we just call it DMARD (pronounced dee-marred) for short. The reason why these drugs are called disease-modifying is because they change the course of the disease and address the underlying issues of inflammation and joint destruction that occur from rheumatoid arthritis.

Whereas Tylenol and ibuprofen are just temporary band-aids to cover up joint pain but don't do much to target the autoimmune process, DMARDs actually stop the vicious cycle of inflammation long-term to produce long-standing protection for the joints.

Commonly used DMARD medications

Methotrexate (Trexall or Rheumatrex)
Leflunomide (Arava)
Sulfasalazine (Azulfidine)
Hydroxychloroquine (Plaquenil)
Azathioprine (Imuran)

What are the benefits of taking a DMARD medication?

The main idea behind starting a DMARD medication is to reduce the joint pain and swelling that causes so much suffering for RA patients. DMARDs also help to improve the function of the joints and have a <u>preventive</u> effect in protecting the joints against deformities and erosions that occur in the structure of the joints.

In the long-term, DMARDs help preserve the integrity and functionality of the joints and prevent joint crippling and disability.

How do DMARD medications work in my body?

After being absorbed through the digestive tract, DMARD medications are broken down by the liver into their active components. They inhibit certain enzymes in the body that immune cells rely on to reproduce and proliferate.

By slowing down the proliferation of the white blood cells in the body, there is decreased production of inflammatory factors and antibodies that lead to the immune system's attack on the joints and other tissues. The result is decreased overall inflammation with improvements in joint pain and swelling.

Further details about each individual DMARD's mechanism of action in the body will be discussed in upcoming sections.

Do DMARDs suppress my immune system?

Yes, they do. In fact, since rheumatoid arthritis is primarily a problem with the body's immune system being overactive, nearly all of the medications used to treat RA are in the immunosuppressant category. This sounds scary to be messing around with the body's immune system, especially during a pandemic when people are getting sick more easily.

A way to think of it is that the immune system has been inappropriately turned on overdrive to damage the body's own tissues, and the medications are meant to tone the immune system back down to normal levels. Like a broken faucet that can't turn itself off and is gushing water when it's not supposed to, the immune system needs help in being turned down. This does require a high degree of consideration and close monitoring for potential side effects, but most patients taking immunosuppressant medications are doing just fine.

Believe it or not, I have had patients, even elderly ones, taking multiple DMARDs together when they contracted the COVID-19 infection, and they just reported mild "cold" or "sinus" symptoms. I'm not saying this is the case for everyone, and patients who are taking immunosuppressant medications should still be extra cautious, but the degree of immunosuppression isn't as severe as you might think. Most of my patients say they haven't noticed catching the cold or flu more easily than before. The immune system is still able to fight off most infections effectively.

How can I tell if a DMARD medication is really working?

When a DMARD starts working, you would have a noticeable reduction in joint pain and swelling. You would also notice an improvement in morning joint stiffness and body stiffness throughout the day.

In the field of rheumatology, we target a "low disease activity level," which means that the arthritis is in remission and there's less of a chance of flares and joint damage in the future. In measuring disease activity level, we mainly consider the number of swollen or painful joints, the patient's overall functioning, and the level of difficulty in participating in activities of daily living and other tasks.

For example, the RAPID-3 is a scoring system used to determine whether a patient's symptoms are in low disease activity or not. Some rheumatologists use the RAPID-3 scoring system at office visits to determine whether a patient is responding well to a treatment or not. The score is tracked over time to determine a patient's trend in inflammatory levels.

How long does it take for a DMARD to start working?

Unfortunately, it can take up to 2-3 months for a DMARD medication to build up to therapeutic levels in the body. This is a long and difficult period of time to wait for someone who is suffering from severe joint pain every day!

While waiting for a DMARD to start working, your rheumatologist may discuss with you the possibility of being on a temporary steroid taper such as prednisone to alleviate symptoms. Later on, the steroid will be tapered off by your rheumatologist, and the DMARD would remain in place as the long-standing treatment. This is a way to overcome the initial hurdle of waiting for a DMARD to start working. Steroids are discussed more in an upcoming section.

Do I have to take DMARDs long-term? Do I have to take them for the rest of my life?

Typically, patients do take DMARDs as a lifelong treatment, unless they experience no improvement from the treatment or if they start having side effects. If the medication isn't bothering you very much, other than the inconvenience of remembering to take a medication on a regular basis, it is usually recommended to continue the same therapy so that the inflammation doesn't come back.

Some patients have felt better after taking a DMARD and stop taking it because they don't feel like they need it anymore, only to experience a flare or exacerbation of their arthritis again.

What are potential side effects of DMARD medications?

The most commonly reported side effects of the DMARD medications are related to the gastrointestinal tract. Patients have experienced nausea, stomach upset, or diarrhea. This could range from mild queasiness that is temporary and goes away after a few doses, to severe nausea and vomiting and inability to tolerate the medication at all.

It's difficult to predict which patients will respond in what way. If you tend to have a sensitive stomach, it's possible you may have more stomach upset than others, but we wouldn't know unless we tried the medication.

Usually, insurance mandates that at least one DMARD medication such as methotrexate is trialed before it would approve coverage of other medications, which can put patients and providers in a bind at times.

More severe side effects of DMARDs would be an elevation in liver enzymes or low blood cell counts. For this reason, labs are usually required for monitoring of these medications every three months. Potential side effects of each DMARD are covered in more detail under individual sections below.

Why are some people scared or hesitant to take a DMARD medication?

The top reason I have heard from my patients after they read about methotrexate on the internet is that it is also used as a chemotherapy drug. The word chemotherapy sounds scary to people, and this is understandable. Some might imagine that they will become a cancer patient who has lost all their hair and is wearing a wig, but this is rarely the case.

It is true that methotrexate, used in much higher doses and with a different drug regimen, is a chemotherapy treatment for certain types of cancers. However, in the field of rheumatology, we are using it in much smaller doses and for a different purpose. We are not using it at high doses to kill off rapidly-dividing cancer cells, but rather at mild doses to regulate an overactive immune system.

Other reasons why some might be fearful of DMARD medications goes back to the idea that it suppresses the immune system to a certain degree or that it might cause unpleasant or dangerous side effects. The truth is that no one can really force you to take a medication that you don't feel comfortable putting in your body. If you have concerns about taking a DMARD medication, certainly share them with your rheumatologist.

How do I know if taking a DMARD medication is worth the risk to me?

Any medication we take (or anything we do in life for that matter) has risks and benefits associated with it. The risks of taking a medication should feel worthwhile to you for the benefit you are receiving. I have had some patients who feel that the risks of taking medications outweigh the potential benefit of alleviating their joint pain and other arthritis symptoms. These patients try to manage their symptoms with the anti-inflammatory diet and holistic methods alone (discussed in other chapters), and everyone's individual beliefs should be respected.

In illustrating risks versus benefits to my patients, I often share the analogy of driving. I personally have some fear of driving because of a bad car accident that I was in as a child with my parents. One of the riskiest things we do every day is driving. Even if you're an excellent driver with a good record, a bad driver or a drunk driver on the road could hit you and cause an injury.

Why do most people still drive then if the rate of car accidents is so high? Because they have places to be, like dropping their kids off at school or going to work. They have accepted the risk of driving for the benefit of having a convenient mode of transportation. I still drive every day and even go on long road trips for vacations even though I feel nervous about driving long-distance, accepting the risk of being on the road for the ability and freedom to travel. The same is true for immunosuppressant medications—weigh the risks and benefits and see if it's worth it to you.

Financial investment risks are also analogous to medication-related risks. As my financial advisor puts it, there's always a possibility that you could invest money and lose it if the economy crashes. "It's possible, but it's not probable" that the risk of investing wasn't worth it in the end.

All we can do is make the most well-educated decision with the knowledge we have today. I think the same concept is applicable to medications that we take and potential side effects we might experience.

When do I stop taking a DMARD medication?

A DMARD is stopped if a patient has a side effect or intolerance of the medication, or if the medication is tried and no improvement is seen in symptoms. For example, if there is severe stomach upset or diarrhea, then the medication could be stopped.

If liver enzymes trend up and no other reasons are found for the change in labs, then rheumatologists usually consider stopping or lowering the dose of the DMARD.

Could I experiment with reducing the dose of my DMARD medication if I feel that my symptoms have been doing well?

A lot of people are wondering if they can reduce the number of medications and pills that they're currently taking. Most of my patients say that they would rather not take a medication if they don't have to, which is true for everyone. Most people would say that less medication, or no medication, is certainly preferred over taking anything at all. I believe in the "lowest effective dose," which means the least medication possible in exchange for a good control of symptoms and a good quality of life.

You could discuss tapering down on the dose of your DMARD medication with your rheumatologist if you would like to. It's possible that your arthritis would flare or symptoms may worsen, and it's also possible that you could do just fine.

In the case that your symptoms do worsen, you could just go back up on the dose again. Typically, there isn't a resistance that your body can develop against DMARD medications, but it will take time to feel better again because the medications take some time to build up to therapeutic levels.

What if I can't tolerate DMARDs or if I have too many side effects?

The good news is that we have a lot of options for treating rheumatoid arthritis these days. If you have given one or two of these DMARD medications a solid trial and it really isn't working out for you, you can move on to the next option. Discuss with your rheumatologist which options would be the best to try next.

Can I receive vaccines while taking a DMARD medication?

Yes, you can receive any vaccine that is an <u>inactivated</u> vaccine—such as the flu shot, new shingles shot, and other inactive ones. Avoid <u>live vaccines</u> such as the flu nasal mist and the measles/mumps/rubella vaccine.

Will DMARDs blunt my immune system's response to vaccines?

There is some evidence that the immune system doesn't respond as well to vaccinations while under the influence of immunosuppressants. If you want to maximize and optimize your immune system's response to a vaccine—for example the COVID-19 vaccine—you could try stopping your immunosuppressant medication temporarily before receiving the vaccine, and then restart it later.

Vaccines will be discussed more in chapter 9, "Navigating rheumatoid arthritis during the COVID-19 pandemic." Next, we will discuss each DMARD in more detail.

METHOTREXATE
(*also known as Trexall or Rheumatrex*)

How long has methotrexate been used for rheumatoid arthritis?

In 1985, scientists discovered that methotrexate relieves joint pain, swelling, and other symptoms in patients with rheumatoid arthritis. It is now widely used as a first-line therapy worldwide for the treatment of rheumatoid arthritis, as well as other autoimmune diseases such as psoriatic arthritis, juvenile arthritis, lupus, and a number of other ones.

Is methotrexate used for anything other than rheumatoid arthritis?

Methotrexate was first produced in 1947 and was originally used to treat cancer. In high doses, it is effective for the treatment of a number of cancers, including breast cancer, head and neck cancers, leukemia, lymphoma, lung cancer, osteosarcoma, bladder cancer, and others.

Methotrexate is on the World Health Organization's List of Essential Medicines, which is a list of the most effective medications that are needed in a healthcare system. In 2019, it was reported to be the 111th most prescribed medication in the United States with more than five million prescriptions.

Methotrexate for autoimmune diseases is taken in lower doses than it is for cancer. Low dose methotrexate is considered a safe and well-tolerated medication in the treatment of autoimmune diseases.

How does methotrexate work?

Methotrexate inhibits an enzyme in the body called "dihydrofolate reductase." This enzyme is involved with producing purines, which is one of the components of DNA. The rapidly dividing immune cells in the body, such as B and T cells, rely heavily on this enzyme and on purines for proliferation and production of inflammatory markers. Without this enzyme, the immune cells cannot proliferate as quickly as usual, and they cannot produce as much inflammation as they would in the autoimmune process.

Methotrexate also causes an increase in "adenosine" within the body. Adenosine inhibits the action of inflammatory cells in the body and has some additional anti-inflammatory properties of its own.

How long does it take for methotrexate to take effect?

As noted before, it takes about 3 months on average for DMARD medications to build up to therapeutic levels. Some patients feel a difference sooner than that, and some say it takes longer.

Patients usually take a steroid taper temporarily while waiting for the medication to start working.

Mechanism of Action

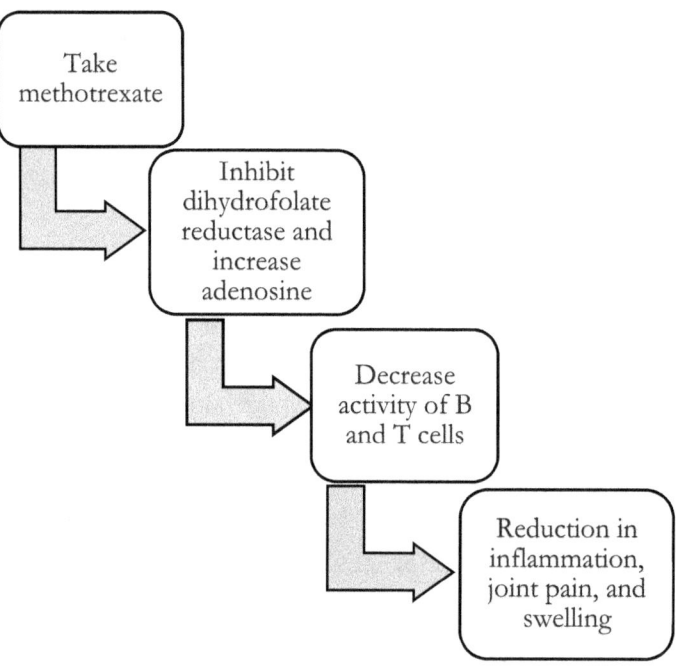

What are the most common side effects of methotrexate?

The side effects of methotrexate can be categorized into minor side effects and major ones. The minor side effects are the more common ones—patients can report feeling tired or having brain fog for a day or two after taking methotrexate. They can have more canker sores or oral ulcers.
Methotrexate can cause stomach upset, nausea, vomiting, or diarrhea, just like any tablet can.

I would say about 50% of my patients don't report any side effects from methotrexate at all. About 25% of patients report that the fatigue or stomach upset from methotrexate are tolerable or temporary, while the other 25% say that they can't take methotrexate anymore because of intolerable side effects.

Another common side effect from methotrexate is that it can cause liver enzyme elevation. For this reason, we check bloodwork every three months when a patient is on methotrexate. Liver enzyme elevation is seen more commonly in patients with fatty liver disease.

Other potential side effects may include hair loss, sensitivity to sunlight exposure, or flu-like symptoms.

What are rare side effects of methotrexate?

In rare cases, methotrexate can cause liver toxicity that is worse than just mildly elevated liver enzymes. When it was first used from the 1940s to the 1980s, cirrhosis of the liver was a feared complication of methotrexate and some patients even got liver biopsies done to be on the safe side. Nowadays, with routine lab monitoring, any liver abnormalities can be caught early on and the medication can be stopped without further issues if there's a high level of concern.

Methotrexate could also cause low blood cell counts, which is another reason regular blood work is done every 3 months. A rare side effect of methotrexate is pulmonary fibrosis, which causes shortness of breath and a chronic dry cough. It usually takes many years of using methotrexate for pulmonary fibrosis to occur in the lungs, and this is rare.

I have seen a couple cases of severe methotrexate toxicity when patients are in the hospital after methotrexate builds up to dangerous levels in the blood. This is rare, but methotrexate toxicity can happen if the kidneys don't work properly and methotrexate builds up too high in the system rather than being eliminated through the kidneys like usual.

Toxicity can also happen if patients are taking the wrong dose of methotrexate (taking it every day instead of only once per week, which is discussed next). Methotrexate toxicity usually causes a severe painful rash on the skin and sores in the mouth, as well as liver problems.

Potential side effects of methotrexate

Nausea, vomiting
Stomach pain or upset
Soft stools or diarrhea
Fatigue or brain fog
Low blood cell counts
Elevated liver enzymes
Canker sores in the mouth

How is methotrexate taken?

Methotrexate is only supposed to be taken <u>once a week</u>! On numerous occasions, this has caused confusion with patients. I usually tell patients in person at their appointments, write it down for them on a piece of paper, and also put it on the prescription bottle so they don't get confused. Some patients are still confused about how to take methotrexate.

A tip is that you can pick a day that is convenient for you, such as a Saturday, or any day that you're not working and won't be too busy. Do not take methotrexate again until the following week. If you take methotrexate every single day, you will become very sick and experience a lot of side effects.

Methotrexate comes as little tablets. Each tablet is 2.5 mg of methotrexate. A typical starting dose is four tablets once per week, which equals 10 mg once per week. The dose can be titrated up slowly over time, if tolerated. The maximum dose for adults is usually eight tablets once per week, which equals 20 mg once per week.

Methotrexate dosing

	Number of tablets once per week	Equivalent amount per week
Starting dose	4	10 mg
Medium dose	6	15 mg
Maximum dose	8	20 mg

Why do I have to take folic acid with methotrexate?

Methotrexate inhibits production of a vitamin called folic acid in the body. Without folic acid, you could experience more canker sores in the mouth or more nausea. Thus, a folic acid vitamin has to be given as a supplement every day so that these side effects do not occur from depletion of folic acid in the body as a result of taking methotrexate.

Folic acid is usually taken as a 1 mg tablet every day. It is written as a prescription that goes along with methotrexate, but some patients say that they can find an over-the-counter folic acid vitamin that is cheaper than the prescription form.

It doesn't matter which version you get, as long as you are taking 1 mg or higher of folic acid every day.

The amount of folic acid stays the same even if the dose of methotrexate changes. Some patients take a higher dose of folic acid, such as 2 mg every day, if they experience side effects like oral ulcers.

Can anything be done to reduce the side effects of methotrexate?

If you're experiencing stomach upset or nausea with taking all the tablets of methotrexate at once, you could try splitting the dose between morning and evening. For example, if you're on the four tablets per week dose, you could take two tablets in the morning and two tablets in the evening rather than all four tablets at once. As long as you're taking all the tablets on the same day once per week, it is the correct dosing.

Taking methotrexate with food also helps with stomach upset and nausea. If methotrexate makes you feel tired after taking it, try taking it in the evening before you go to bed. And again, some patients take a higher dose of folic acid, such as 2 mg every day, if they have side effects like oral ulcers.

Does methotrexate come in forms other than tablets?

Methotrexate also comes as an injectable form, also known as "Rasuvo" or "Otrexup." This is a liquid formulation of methotrexate that comes in a syringe and can be injected under the skin, usually in the lower abdomen or the upper thighs, similar to an insulin injection.

The injectable form of methotrexate can be used if a patient has trouble with stomach upset after taking the pills, or if there is a digestive tract problem that causes an inability to absorb medications normally (for example, Crohn's disease or a previous bowel surgery). The subcutaneous injection has good bioavailability, which means that it reaches therapeutic levels in the body reliably. Patients can still experience the side effects, such as the nausea, fatigue, or liver enzyme elevation with the injectable form of methotrexate.

Does methotrexate require routine bloodwork to be done?

Initially, labs are done once a month until a stable dose of methotrexate is reached. Then, labs are required to be drawn every three months while taking methotrexate.

Your rheumatologist will usually monitor two labs, a CBC and a CMP. The CBC is a "complete blood count" and will make sure your white blood cells, red blood cells, and platelets are staying healthy while taking methotrexate. The CMP is a "complete metabolic profile" and will check if your liver, kidneys, and electrolytes are normal while taking methotrexate.

How do I protect my liver while taking methotrexate?

Upon starting methotrexate, we recommend that patients reduce their alcohol consumption to about three drinks of alcohol per week or less. Since methotrexate is metabolized by the liver, drinking too much alcohol could cause stress on the liver and cause liver enzymes to increase.

A handful of patients don't feel that it's realistic to reduce their alcohol use to three drinks per week or less. For example, I have a patient who is in sales and has to "wine and dine" his clients as part of his job. I also have a patient who drinks about a bottle of wine per day and has always done that throughout his adult life. If you don't feel like it's realistic or possible to limit your alcohol intake to a certain level, please let your rheumatologist know so that alternatives can be discussed.

Is methotrexate safe during pregnancy and breastfeeding?

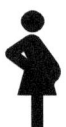

Definitely not. Methotrexate is known to be teratogenic, which means that it will cause harm to a fetus developing in the womb and malformations to occur in a baby. It should also be avoided during breastfeeding.

Women of childbearing age are required to be on reliable contraception before starting methotrexate. Men should also notify their rheumatologist if they are trying to conceive with their partner. A small amount of methotrexate may enter the ejaculatory fluid, which could affect female partners.

Please discuss family planning with your rheumatologist. Methotrexate has a long half-life and stays in the body for up to 3-6 months after stopping it, so any women who would like to start a family should stop taking methotrexate many months ahead of time before attempting to conceive.

Is there any reason I should not take methotrexate?

Patients with liver cirrhosis or severe kidney impairment, such as patients on dialysis, should not take methotrexate. Patients with active hepatitis B and C infections should not take methotrexate.

Your rheumatologist will check hepatitis B and C labs prior to starting methotrexate. Women who are pregnant or are attempting to conceive should not start methotrexate.

Drug interactions with methotrexate

Acitretin
Meloxicam
Trimethoprim
Digoxin
Dapsone

What if I can't tolerate methotrexate or if I have too many side effects?

The good news is that we have many options for treating rheumatoid arthritis these days. I have some patients who swear by methotrexate as a miracle drug and wouldn't consider taking anything else for their arthritis, and other patients who really don't like methotrexate at all.

If you have given methotrexate a solid trial and it really isn't working out for you, you can move on to the next option, which could be another DMARD medication, a biologic, or a JAK inhibitor (discussed more in upcoming chapters). Discuss with your rheumatologist which options would be the best to try next.

LEFLUNOMIDE
(also known as Arava)

How long has leflunomide been used for rheumatoid arthritis?

Leflunomide was approved by the FDA for use in rheumatoid arthritis in 1998. Leflunomide can be considered a "cousin" of methotrexate since they work in similar ways (but on different enzymes in the body) and can have similar side effects.

Is leflunomide used for anything other than rheumatoid arthritis?

Leflunomide can also be used to treat psoriatic arthritis. It is still being researched for use in other autoimmune conditions such as lupus and lupus nephritis.

How does leflunomide work?

Leflunomide inhibits an enzyme in the body called "dihydro-orotate dehydrogenase." This enzyme is involved with producing pyrimidines, which is one of the components of DNA.

The rapidly dividing immune cells in the body, such as B and T cells, rely heavily on this enzyme and on pyrimidines for proliferation and production of inflammatory markers. Without this enzyme, the immune cells cannot proliferate as quickly as usual, and they cannot produce as much inflammation as they would in the autoimmune process.

Mechanism of Action

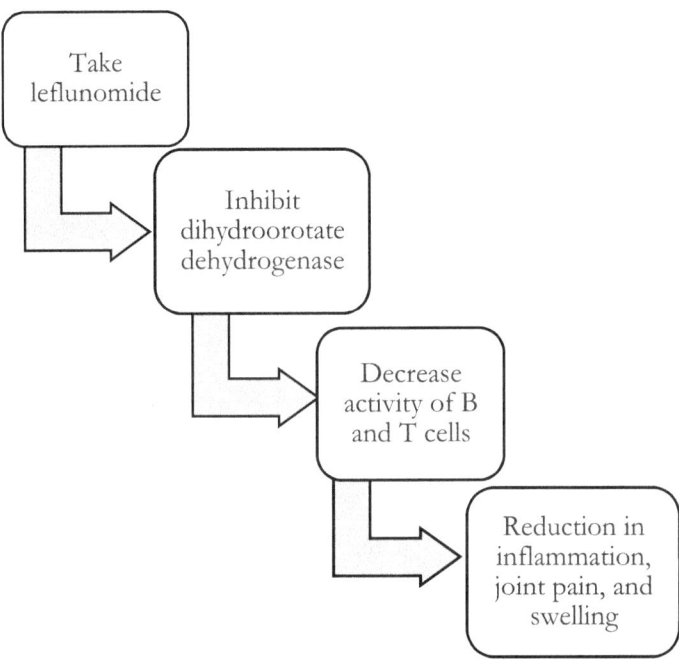

How long does it take for leflunomide to take effect?

As noted above, it takes about 3 months on average for any DMARD medication to build up to therapeutic levels. Some patients feel a difference sooner than that, and some say it takes longer.

What are the most common side effects of leflunomide?

The side effects of leflunomide are similar to the side effects of methotrexate. The minor side effects are the more common ones—patients can report feeling tired or having brain fog after taking leflunomide. They can have more canker sores or oral ulcers. Leflunomide can cause stomach upset, nausea, vomiting, or diarrhea, just like any tablet can.

I would say that about 50% of my patients don't report any side effects from leflunomide at all. About 25% of patients report that the fatigue, stomach upset, or diarrhea from leflunomide are tolerable or temporary, whether the other 25% say that they can't take leflunomide anymore because of intolerable side effects.

Another common side effect from leflunomide is that it can cause liver enzyme elevation. For this reason, we check bloodwork every three months when a patient is on leflunomide. Liver enzyme elevation is seen more commonly in patients with fatty liver disease.

Other side effects may include hair loss, sensitivity to sunlight exposure, or flu-like symptoms.

What are rare side effects of leflunomide?

Just like with methotrexate, leflunomide can cause liver toxicity that is worse than just mildly elevated liver enzymes in rare cases. With routine lab monitoring, any liver abnormalities can be caught early on and the medication can be stopped without further issues.

Leflunomide can worsen high blood pressure in some cases, so blood pressure is checked routinely at each appointment during therapy. Leflunomide could also cause low blood cell counts, which is another reason regular blood work is done every 3 months.

A rare side effect of leflunomide is a lung condition called interstitial pneumonitis, which causes shortness of breath and a chronic dry cough. It usually takes many years of using leflunomide for interstitial pneumonitis to occur in the lungs, and a study done in Japan showed that only eighty cases were reported between 2003 and 2006.

Potential side effects of leflunomide

Nausea, vomiting
Stomach pain or upset
Soft stools or diarrhea
Fatigue or brain fog
Low blood cell counts
Elevated liver enzymes
High blood pressure
Weight loss

How is leflunomide taken?

Leflunomide is taken as one tablet per day. The starting dose is 10 mg daily, which can be increased up to the maximum dose of 20 mg daily if needed. There is no injectable form of leflunomide, only the tablet form.

Leflunomide dosing

Starting dose: 10 mg daily
Maximum dose: 20 mg daily

Do I have to take folic acid with leflunomide?

No, leflunomide does not affect the enzyme that lowers folic acid production in the body. Folic acid supplementation is only needed with methotrexate, not with any other DMARD medications.

Can anything be done to reduce the side effects of leflunomide?

If you're experiencing stomach upset or nausea with taking leflunomide, make sure you take it with a meal. If leflunomide makes you feel tired after taking it, try taking it in the evening before you go to bed.

Does leflunomide require routine bloodwork to be done?

Initially, labs are done once a month until a stable dose of leflunomide is reached. Then, labs are required to be drawn every three months while taking leflunomide.

Your rheumatologist will usually monitor two labs, a CBC and a CMP. The CBC is a "complete blood count" and will make sure your white blood cells, red blood cells, and platelets are staying healthy while taking leflunomide. The CMP is a "complete metabolic profile" and will check if your liver, kidneys, and electrolytes are normal while taking leflunomide.

How do I protect my liver while taking leflunomide?

Upon starting leflunomide, we recommend that patients reduce their alcohol consumption to about three drinks of alcohol per week or less. Since leflunomide is metabolized by the liver, drinking too much alcohol could cause stress on the liver and elevated liver enzymes.

Again, if you don't feel like it's possible to limit your alcohol intake to a certain level, please let your rheumatologist know so that alternatives can be discussed.

Is leflunomide safe during pregnancy and breastfeeding?

Definitely not. Leflunomide is known to be teratogenic, which means that it will cause harm to a fetus developing in the womb and malformations to occur. Women of childbearing age are required to be on reliable contraception before starting leflunomide. Avoid leflunomide if you are breastfeeding.

Men should also notify their rheumatologist if they are trying to conceive with their partner. A small amount of leflunomide may enter the ejaculatory fluid, which could affect female partners.

Please discuss family planning with your rheumatologist. Leflunomide has an even longer half-life than methotrexate and stays in the body for up to 6-8 months after stopping it, so any women who would like to start a family should stop taking this medication several months ahead of time before attempting to conceive. If pregnancy accidentally occurs, a detoxification protocol has to take place to eliminate leflunomide more quickly from the body.

Drug interactions with leflunomide

Carvedilol
Phenytoin and fosphenytoin
Warfarin
Tamoxifen
Losartan

Is there any reason I should not take leflunomide?

Patients with liver cirrhosis or severe kidney impairment, such as patients on dialysis, should not take leflunomide.

Patients with active hepatitis B and C infections should not take leflunomide.

Your rheumatologist will check hepatitis B and C labs prior to starting leflunomide. Women who are pregnant or are attempting to conceive should not start leflunomide.

SULFASALAZINE
(also known as Azulfidine)

How long has sulfasalazine been used for rheumatoid arthritis?

Sulfasalazine was approved by the FDA for use in rheumatoid arthritis in 1950. It is another widely used medication for rheumatoid arthritis.

Is sulfasalazine used for anything other than rheumatoid arthritis?

Sulfasalazine is also used to treat inflammatory bowel diseases, such as Crohn's disease or ulcerative colitis, as well as certain types of arthritis that can occur with inflammatory bowel disease. Sulfasalazine can be used for psoriatic arthritis and reactive arthritis as well.

How does sulfasalazine work?

Sulfasalazine is broken down by intestinal bacteria into its active components, "sulfapyridine and 5-aminosalicyclic acid." These active components reduce inflammation in the digestive tract. Although still not completely clear, sulfasalazine exerts systemic anti-inflammatory effects throughout the body as well.

The "leaky gut theory" was discussed in a separate section and hypothesizes that the gut is the primary part of the body where inflammation begins. This concept helps us understand why sulfasalazine reduces inflammation in the entire body by reducing inflammation in the gut.

There is also extensive research that the microbiome of the gut affects the development of rheumatoid arthritis, and targeting the inflammation in the digestive tract is key to controlling inflammation throughout the body.

How long does it take for sulfasalazine to take effect?

As noted above, it takes about 3 months on average for DMARD medications to build up to therapeutic levels. Some patients feel a difference sooner than that, and some say it takes longer.

What are the most common side effects of sulfasalazine?

The most common side effect of sulfasalazine is diarrhea and stomach upset. This can range from soft stools to multiple episodes of watery diarrhea per day, which usually makes patients want to stop taking the medication.

Sulfasalazine can cause low sperm counts in men, which becomes important in young men who want to start a family. The low sperm count is reversible upon stopping sulfasalazine and infertility is temporary.

Mechanism of Action

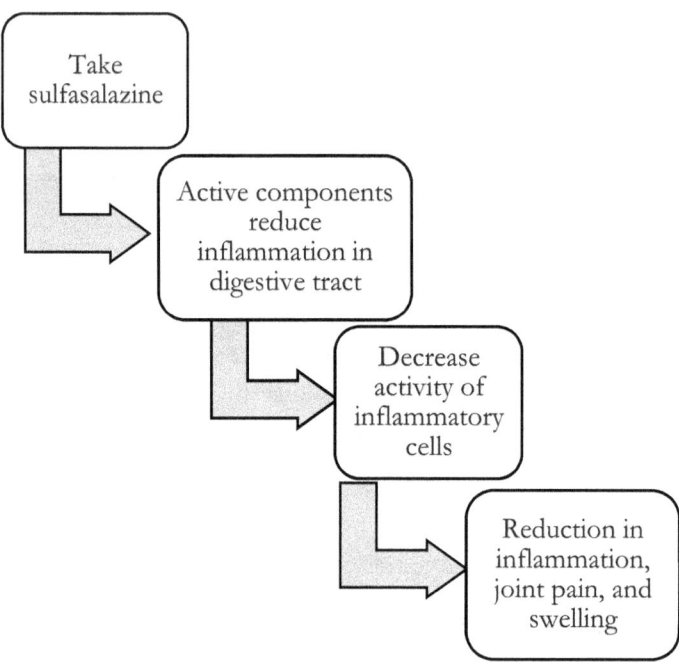

What are rare side effects of sulfasalazine?

In rare cases, sulfasalazine can cause low blood cell counts such as low white blood cell counts or low platelet levels. In patients with a history of G6PD deficiency (enzyme in the body that helps red blood cells function), sulfasalazine can cause hemolytic anemia, which is dangerous. Rheumatologists typically check a patient's G6PD enzyme levels prior to starting sulfasalazine, especially for patients of Mediterranean descent.

Potential side effects of sulfasalazine

Nausea, vomiting
Stomach pain or upset

- Soft stools or diarrhea
- Fatigue
- Low blood cell counts
- Elevated liver enzymes
- Hemolytic anemia with G6PD deficiency
- Sulfa allergy
- Temporary infertility, low sperm counts in men

How is sulfasalazine taken?

Sulfasalazine comes in relatively large tablets and each tablet equals 500 mg. A typical starting dose is 500 mg once daily or twice daily, split between morning and evening. You can start with one tablet per day with a meal to begin with, and increase to twice daily after one week if you're feeling okay. The dose can be slowly titrated up over time if needed.

The dose is usually increased slowly so that the body can get used to the medication and so that side effects like diarrhea and stomach upset can be avoided. There is no injectable form of sulfasalazine, only tablets.

Sulfasalazine dosing

	Morning	Evening
Starting dose	500 mg (1 tablet)	500 mg (1 tablet)
Intermediate dose	1000 mg (2 tablets)	1000 mg (2 tablets)
Maximum dose	1500 mg (3 tablets)	1500 mg (3 tablets)

Can anything be done to reduce the side effects of sulfasalazine?

If you're experiencing stomach upset or nausea with taking sulfasalazine, make sure you take it with a meal. Sulfasalazine also comes in an enteric-coated and delayed-release formulation which usually causes less gastrointestinal side effects. Check to see if your pharmacy carries the delayed-release formulation of sulfasalazine which may be easier on the stomach and digestive tract.

Does sulfasalazine require routine bloodwork to be done?

Initially, labs are done once a month until a stable dose of sulfasalazine is reached. Then, labs are required to be drawn every three months while taking sulfasalazine.

Your rheumatologist will usually monitor two labs, a CBC and a CMP every three months. The CBC is a "complete blood count" and will make sure your white blood cells, red blood cells, and platelets are staying healthy while taking sulfasalazine. The CMP is a "complete metabolic profile" and will check if your liver, kidneys, and electrolytes are normal.

How do I protect my liver while taking sulfasalazine?

Sulfasalazine tends to affect the liver less so than methotrexate or leflunomide. However, we still recommend that patients reduce their alcohol consumption to about three drinks of alcohol per week or less while taking this medication. Since sulfasalazine is also metabolized by the liver, drinking too much alcohol could cause stress on the liver and elevated liver enzymes.

Again, if you don't feel like it's possible to limit your alcohol intake to a certain level, please let your rheumatologist know so that alternatives can be discussed.

Is sulfasalazine safe during pregnancy and breastfeeding?

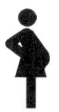

Typically not. Women of childbearing age are required to be on reliable contraception before starting sulfasalazine. Avoid this medication if you are breastfeeding.

Men should also notify their rheumatologist if they are trying to conceive with their partner since sulfasalazine can cause temporary low sperm counts. Please discuss family planning with your rheumatologist before starting sulfasalazine and during therapy.

Drug interactions with sulfasalazine

Ketorolac
Acetazolamide
Atenolol
Captopril
Digoxin

Is there any reason I should not take sulfasalazine?

Patients with sulfa allergies should avoid sulfasalazine. Patients with G6PD deficiency should not take sulfasalazine. Patients with active hepatitis B and C infections should not take sulfasalazine.

Women who are pregnant or are attempting to conceive should not start sulfasalazine. Men who are attempting to start families should not take sulfasalazine.

HYDROXYCHLOROQUINE
(*also known as Plaquenil*)

How long has hydroxychloroquine been used for rheumatoid arthritis?

Hydroxychloroquine is a very old drug and was first approved for use in 1955. It is also on the World Health Organization's list of essential medicines. Surprisingly, its original use was for treatment of malaria.

It was noted that patients taking hydroxychloroquine for malaria experienced an improvement in their autoimmune symptoms, such as joint pain and swelling. There are also ancient writings found from Incan and Mayan civilizations describing a medicine derived from a tree bark that helped with joint pain and other symptoms. This ancient medication is believed to be hydroxychloroquine.

Is hydroxychloroquine used for anything other than rheumatoid arthritis?

Hydroxychloroquine is used to treat a number of autoimmune diseases, the main one being systemic lupus erythematosus and lupus nephritis. Hydroxychloroquine is also sometimes used to treat Sjogren syndrome, scleroderma, dermatomyositis, and other autoimmune diseases.

How does hydroxychloroquine work?

Hydroxychloroquine works in a number of ways to decrease inflammation within the immune system. It works on a component within cells called "lysosomes." By increasing the pH within lysosomes, immune cells produce less inflammatory products such as cytokines.

Hydroxychloroquine also works on "toll-like receptors" within the immune system. Toll-like receptors are part of the innate immune system and activate immune responses and release of inflammatory markers. Inhibiting the toll-like receptors results in a reduction in systemic inflammation.

How long does it take for hydroxychloroquine to take effect?

Hydroxychloroquine is notoriously slow-working since it is the mildest of all the DMARD medications. It can take up to 4-6 months, on average, for hydroxychloroquine to build up to therapeutic levels.

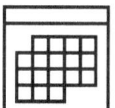

I have had some patients tell me that they take hydroxychloroquine for one week and feel a world of difference. I have also had some patients say that it took 6 months for hydroxychloroquine to start working, or that they never felt anything from it at all. It is usually a medication worth waiting for, because it can exert long-lasting protective effects and doesn't cause many side effects.

What are the most common side effects of hydroxychloroquine?

The most common side effect of hydroxychloroquine is that it can cause stomach upset or nausea. Patients have also reported headaches or dizziness at times.

Mechanism of Action

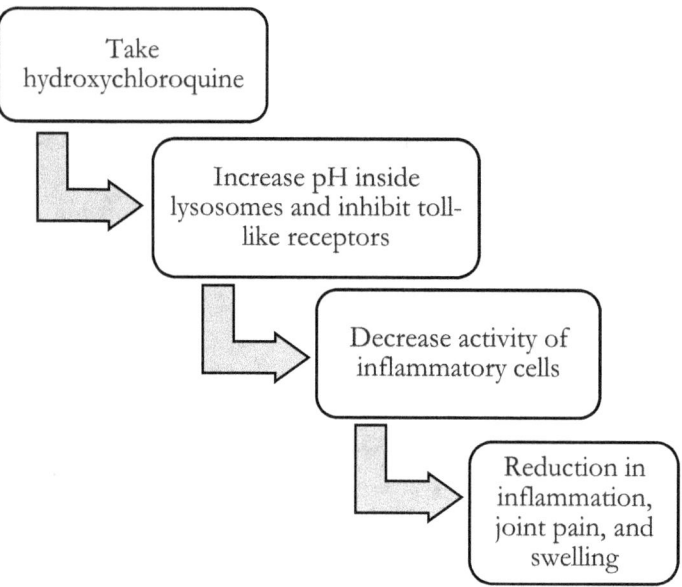

What are rare side effects of hydroxychloroquine?

In rare cases, hydroxychloroquine can affect the retina, which is the "back part" of the eyes. Typically, this can start to occur after about 10-20 years of taking hydroxychloroquine.

Patients are usually scared when they hear that a medication can affect their vision and they worry they might become blind. Blindness is rarely the case—a change in color vision or peripheral vision is more common—but still rare. My colleagues who are eye doctors have told me that they have never or rarely seen a case of hydroxychloroquine-associated retinal toxicity.

Nevertheless, since the eyes are such vital organs, an annual eye examination is recommended. If you tell your eye doctor (optometrist or ophthalmologist) that you are taking hydroxychloroquine, they will do special testing to examine and monitor your eyes. Typically, an eye doctor can see changes occurring in the retina before any symptoms occur. This is why it's so important to have a baseline eye exam upon starting hydroxychloroquine and then stay up-to-date with an annual eye exam every year.

Another rare side effect of hydroxychloroquine is that it can affect the heart. A segment of the heart's electrical rhythm, called the QT interval, can be prolonged with doses of hydroxychloroquine that are too high, or when there are drug interactions between hydroxychloroquine and other cardiac medications. See more about dosing below.

Potential side effects of hydroxychloroquine

Nausea, vomiting
Stomach pain or upset
Soft stools or diarrhea
Retinal toxicity
Rash or skin hyperpigmentation
Sensitivity to sun exposure
Abnormal heart rhythm

How is hydroxychloroquine taken?

Hydroxychloroquine comes in 200 mg tablets. Typically, a person's ideal dose of hydroxychloroquine depends on their weight in kilograms. A safe dose of hydroxychloroquine is specified to be 5 mg per kilogram. Exceeding this dose would result in a higher risk of retinal toxicity for the eyes.

The dose is usually split between morning and evening to prevent stomach upset, but if it doesn't bother the stomach, patients can take two of the 200 mg tablets together if it's easier to remember to take it once a day. There is no injectable form of hydroxychloroquine, only oral tablets.

Hydroxychloroquine dosing

Weight 40 kg or less: 200 mg daily
Weight between 40-80 kg: 300 mg daily
Weight 80 kg or more: 400 mg daily

Can anything be done to reduce the side effects of hydroxychloroquine?

If you're experiencing stomach upset or nausea with taking hydroxychloroquine, make sure you take it with a meal. If you're taking two tablets per day, you could split the tablets between morning and evening or reduce the dose to one tablet per day to see if that's better.

Does hydroxychloroquine require routine bloodwork to be done?

No, hydroxychloroquine does not require blood work to be done at regular intervals. It does not tend to affect blood cell counts, kidney function, or liver enzymes. The only monitoring that is required is the baseline eye exam and then a comprehensive eye exam once per year after that.

How do I protect my eyes while taking hydroxychloroquine?

Staying within the recommended dosage of hydroxychloroquine, which is 5 mg per kilogram, will be safest to reduce the risk of retinal changes. Scheduling a baseline and an annual eye examination will help monitor for any early changes developing in the retina.

Again, retinal damage from hydroxychloroquine is rare, but the eyes are a very important part of our bodies, so extra precautions are taken.

Is hydroxychloroquine safe during pregnancy and breastfeeding?

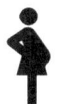

Yes, hydroxychloroquine has been proven to be safe for pregnancy and in breastfeeding. In fact, hydroxychloroquine has been shown to have protective effects for the developing fetus, especially in mothers with lupus (which has been studied extensively).

Hydroxychloroquine does not have to be discontinued before attempting conception or during pregnancy. It is the only DMARD that is known to be safe during pregnancy and breastfeeding.

Is there any reason I should not take hydroxychloroquine?

Tell your rheumatologist if you have any underlying eye conditions such as macular degeneration or retinoschisis. Your eye doctor may need to give permission for you to take hydroxychloroquine with underlying retinal conditions. Eye conditions like glaucoma and cataracts are not affected by hydroxychloroquine, only retinal conditions.

Does hydroxychloroquine have any drug interactions?

Tell your rheumatologist if you are taking tamoxifen, a medication for breast cancer, which has drug interactions with hydroxychloroquine and can increase its toxicity.

Drug interactions with hydroxychloroquine

Tamoxifen
Lefamulin
Amiodarone
Amitriptyline
Levofloxacin

AZATHIOPRINE
(*also known as Imuran*)

How long has azathioprine been used for rheumatoid arthritis?

Azathioprine was approved by the FDA for treatment of rheumatoid arthritis in 1957. It is typically used as a third or fourth-line treatment for rheumatoid arthritis, after the other DMARDs have been tried and don't work well or cause side effects.

Is azathioprine used for anything other than rheumatoid arthritis?

Azathioprine is also used to treat other autoimmune diseases such as lupus nephritis, sarcoidosis, and certain types of vasculitis. It is sometimes used after kidney and organ transplant surgeries to prevent the host's immune system from rejecting the donor's organ.

How does azathioprine work?

Azathioprine is converted to an active form called "6-mercaptopurine" in the body. The active component inhibits production of purines, which is one of the components of DNA.

The rapidly dividing immune cells in the body, such as B and T cells, rely heavily on purines for proliferation and production of inflammatory markers. Due to inhibition of purine production, the immune cells cannot proliferate as quickly as usual, and they cannot produce as much inflammation as they would in the autoimmune process.

How long does it take for azathioprine to take effect?

It takes about 3 months on average for DMARD medications like azathioprine to build up to therapeutic levels. Some patients feel a difference sooner than that, and some say it takes longer.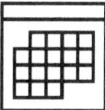

What are the most common side effects of azathioprine?

The side effects of azathioprine are similar to the side effects of methotrexate and leflunomide. Azathioprine can cause stomach upset, nausea, vomiting, or diarrhea, just like any tablet can. Azathioprine can also cause fatigue or rashes.

Another common side effect from azathioprine is that it can cause liver enzyme elevation. For this reason, we check bloodwork every three months when a patient is on azathioprine. Liver enzyme elevation is seen more commonly in patients with fatty liver disease.

Mechanism of Action

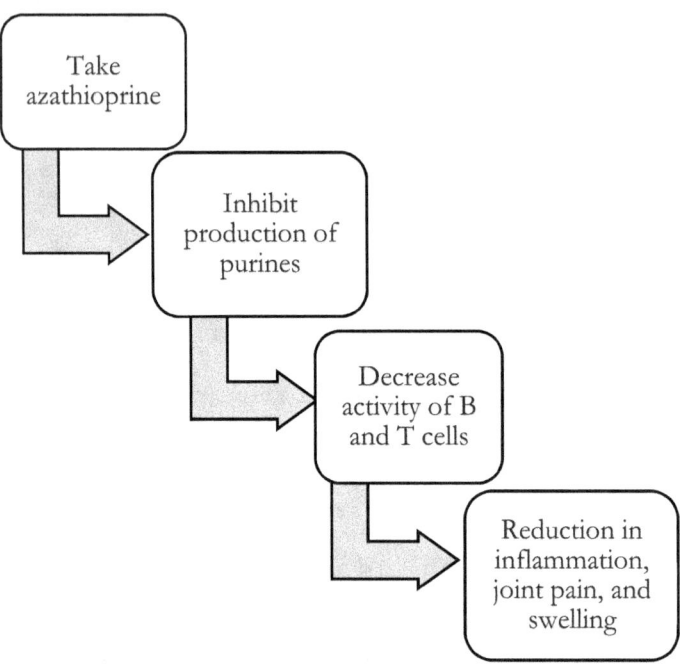

What are rare side effects of azathioprine?

In rare cases, azathioprine can cause bone marrow suppression and very low blood cell counts. This would pose a risk of serious infections.

Rheumatologists also check a "TPMT level" before starting azathioprine. TPMT is an enzyme in your body that processes azathioprine and allows it to be eliminated from the body instead of building up. Some people have a genetic deficiency of the TPMT enzyme and cannot process azathioprine normally.

If azathioprine builds up too much in the body, it can cause a toxic syndrome with symptoms of rash, fever, low blood cell counts, liver damage, and other symptoms.

Potential side effects of azathioprine

Nausea, vomiting
Stomach pain or upset
Soft stools or diarrhea
Fatigue
Low blood cell counts
Elevated liver enzymes
Increased toxicity with TPMT deficiency

How is azathioprine taken?

Azathioprine usually comes in 50 mg tablets. Patients can start with one tablet per day and titrate up slowly on the dose as tolerated. The maximum dose is usually 150 mg daily. There is no injectable form of azathioprine, only oral tablets.

Azathioprine dosing

Starting dose	50 mg daily
Medium dose	50 mg twice daily
Maximum dose	50 mg three times per day

Do I have to take folic acid with azathioprine?

No, azathioprine does not affect the enzyme that lowers folic acid production in the body. Folic acid supplementation is only needed with methotrexate, not with other DMARD medications.

Can anything be done to reduce the side effects of azathioprine?

If you're experiencing stomach upset or nausea with taking azathioprine, make sure you take it with a meal. If azathioprine makes you feel tired after taking it, try taking it in the evening before you go to bed. Your rheumatologist will check TPMT prior to initiation of azathioprine.

Does azathioprine require routine bloodwork to be done?

Initially, labs are done once a month until a stable dose of azathioprine is reached. Then, labs are required to be drawn every three months while taking azathioprine.

Your rheumatologist will usually monitor two labs, a CBC and a CMP. The CBC is a "complete blood count" and will make sure your white blood cells, red blood cells, and platelets are staying healthy while taking azathioprine. The CMP is a "complete metabolic profile" and will check if your liver, kidneys, and electrolytes are normal while taking azathioprine.

How do I protect my liver while taking azathioprine?

Upon starting azathioprine, we recommend that patients reduce their alcohol consumption to about three drinks of alcohol per week or less. Since azathioprine is metabolized by the liver, drinking too much alcohol could cause stress on the liver and elevated liver enzymes.

Again, if you don't feel like it's possible to limit your alcohol intake to a certain level, please let your rheumatologist know so that alternatives can be discussed.

Is azathioprine safe during pregnancy and breastfeeding?

No, azathioprine is known to be teratogenic, which means that it will cause harm and malformations to a fetus developing in the womb. Women of childbearing age are required to be on reliable contraception before starting azathioprine. Azathioprine is only taken in pregnancy if there are no other suitable alternatives and the autoimmune disease is severely flaring up or causing organ damage to the mother.

Please discuss family planning with your rheumatologist. Azathioprine can stay in the body for up to 3-4 months after stopping it, so any women who would like to start a family should stop taking this medication many months ahead of time before attempting to conceive. Avoid azathioprine if you are breastfeeding.

Does azathioprine have any drug interactions?

Azathioprine has some important drug interactions with certain gout medications. Do not take azathioprine with allopurinol or febuxostat (Uloric) due to increased risk of toxicity.

Drug interactions with azathioprine

Allopurinol
Febuxostat (Uloric)
Tacrolimus
Glatiramer
Everolimus

Is there any reason I should not take azathioprine?

Patients with the TPMT enzyme deficiency should not take azathioprine because it will build up to toxic levels. Patients with liver cirrhosis or severe kidney impairment, such as patients on dialysis, should not take azathioprine.

Patients with active hepatitis B and C infections should not take azathioprine. Your rheumatologist will check hepatitis B and C labs prior to starting leflunomide. Women who are pregnant or are attempting to conceive should not start azathioprine.

SUMMARY OF DMARD TREATMENTS

	Liver monitoring	Blood cell count monitoring	Eye monitoring	Folic acid supplementation	Safe during pregnancy and breastfeeding	Alcohol restriction
Methotrexate	✓	✓		✓		✓
Leflunomide	✓	✓				✓
Sulfasalazine	✓	✓				✓
Hydroxychloroquine			✓		✓	
Azathioprine	✓	✓				✓

Final Thoughts on DMARDs

How long do I have to try a DMARD before considering switching to another medication?

Patients usually try a DMARD for 3 months or longer before switching to another medication. If they experience a side effect, switching to a new medication usually occurs sooner.

What if I can't tolerate DMARDs or if I have too many side effects?

The good news is that we have many options for treating rheumatoid arthritis these days. If you have given one or two of these medications a solid trial and it really isn't working out for you, you can move on to the next option. Discuss with your rheumatologist which options would be the best to try next.

Financial and Insurance Considerations: are DMARD medications affordable?

Since DMARDs are older medications that have been around for a long time, they are typically very affordable and low-cost. They usually cost around $20-30 per month, sometimes less, depending on your insurance plan.

The only time I have seen a DMARD medication cost a lot of money is when a patient had a really high insurance deductible at the beginning of the year, and any of his/her medications would have been expensive at that time until he/she paid through the deductible.

Case scenarios

These case scenarios are illustrations of journeys that different patients may experience, which are loosely based on the paths that some of my patients have taken with DMARD medications. Names have been changed for anonymity.

Case 1

Kevin was extremely hesitant to start medications to treat his rheumatoid arthritis after diagnosis. He was never a medicine-taker and barely even took an ibuprofen or Tylenol once in a while for headaches. He read some scary things about methotrexate online and overall didn't like that these medications were going to suppress his immune system during a pandemic.

However, his rheumatoid arthritis was starting to interfere with his work as a chef and he was worried about the use of his hands in the long run. He started taking methotrexate and felt better after 1-2 months or so. He was surprised that he never actually experienced any side effects from the medication such as nausea or stomach upset.

Since he still had some residual symptoms after being on the starting dose of methotrexate for 3 months, he and his rheumatologist discussed increasing his dose of methotrexate to a medium dose. He felt resolution of his symptoms on this dose and his labs were done every 3 months without any abnormalities detected. He continued taking methotrexate as a long-standing treatment without issues.

Case 2

Susan tried taking methotrexate, but it caused elevated liver enzymes after 6 months of taking it. The methotrexate also made her feel nauseated and tired for about 1-2 days after taking it on Sundays. Especially with her history of fatty liver disease, she and her rheumatologist didn't want to add any other medications that would put an additional stress on her liver.

Susan opted to take one of the injectable biologics instead, which ended up working well and didn't cause any side effects.

Case 3

Pam took methotrexate without any side effects and was able to titrate up to the maximum dose of 8 tablets once per week with folic acid. She felt that even on the maximum dose of methotrexate, it was only partially helpful and she continued to have some symptoms of joint pain, stiffness, and swelling. She still had trouble gardening and getting chores done around the house.

Her rheumatologist suggested adding the biologic Humira at this point, but Pam has a fear of needles and didn't like the sound of injecting herself at home on an every-other-week basis. Thus, she opted to take the triple DMARD therapy, which is a combination of methotrexate, sulfasalazine, and hydroxychloroquine. Even though it was a lot of pills to take, she felt more comfortable with this strategy rather than an injection.

Reflection questions: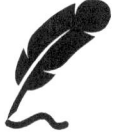

1. What aspects of DMARD treatments seem like they would be a good fit with you?

2. What aspects of DMARD treatments seem concerning to you?

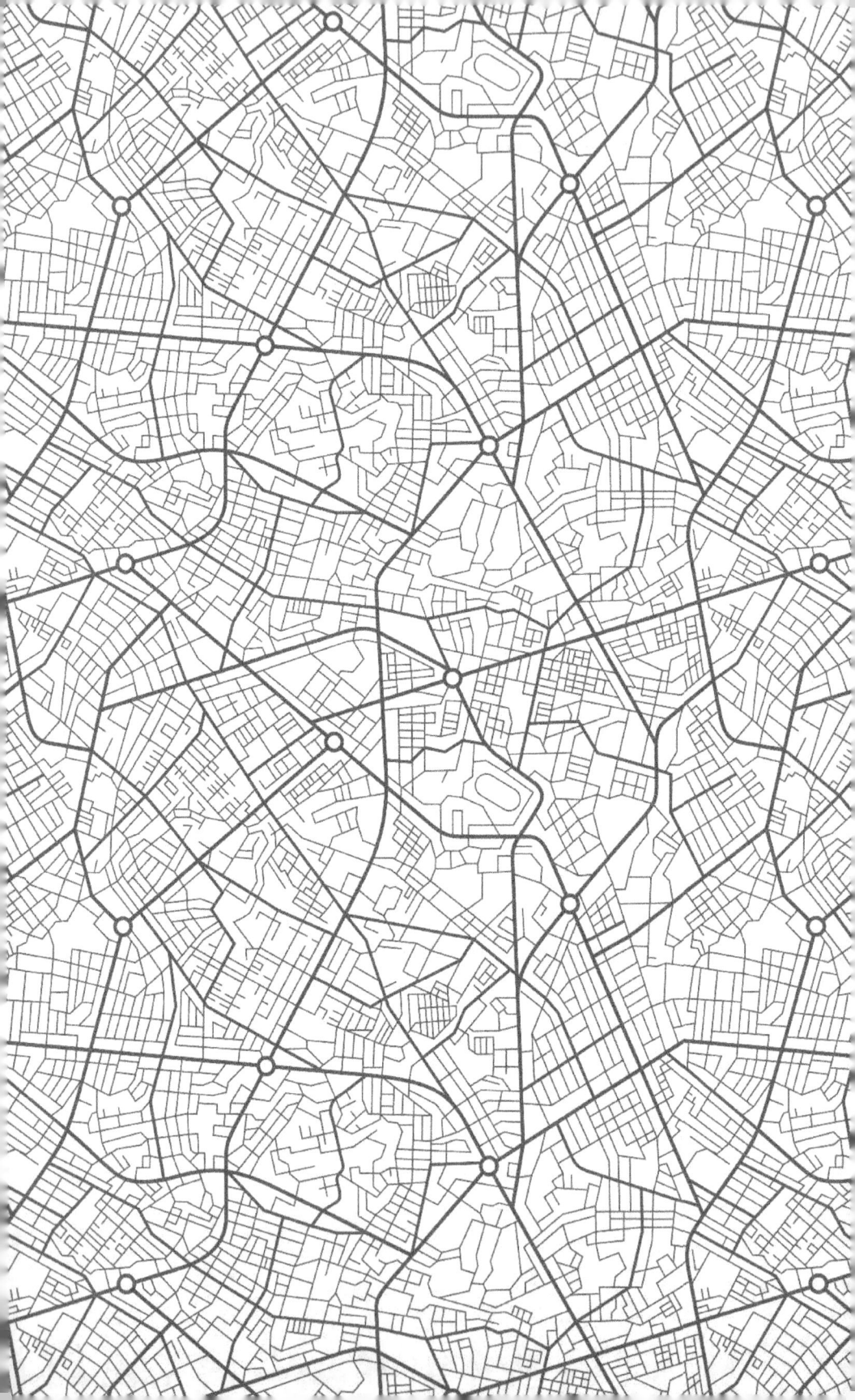

CHAPTER 4
NAVIGATING BIOLOGIC TREATMENTS

ADVANCEMENTS IN RHEUMATOID ARTHRITIS TREATMENT

How are rheumatoid arthritis treatments different now than they were in the past?

Whereas older RA treatments were DMARDs that targeted general inflammation and enzymes to slow immune cell proliferation, the newer biologics are targeted towards very specific inflammatory molecules in the immune system. You can think of DMARDs as a police force to slow down the overall crime in an area, whereas biologics are highly trained assassins tailored to take down a very specific target, like a mafia boss.

As an example, TNF is an inflammatory marker in the body that has been shown to be elevated in rheumatoid arthritis. The overactive immune cells produce large quantities of TNF when a patient has rheumatoid arthritis. By using a biologic to block the TNF molecule and make it inactive, TNF can no longer cause inflammation, joint pain, and damage.

What are examples of newer treatments for rheumatoid arthritis?

The newer treatments are biologics like Humira or Enbrel. They are called "biologics" because they are created from antibodies from living organisms, such as antibodies from the immune systems of humans or animals such as a rabbit or a mouse. These antibodies target molecules like TNF, or act as a decoy receptor, to block it from reaching its destination.

Do treatments come in forms other than tablets or pills?

Biologics are injectable medications rather than tablets or pills. An injection can be taken once per week or every other week (sometimes even longer), rather than taking a pill every day.

Injections can sound scary because they involve needles, but biologics usually come in an autoinjector pen, similar to an "Epi-pen." The needle is very small and typically hidden within the tube. With the press of a button, the medication is usually injected into the lower abdomen or upper thighs. Some of the biologics don't come in an autoinjector and may look more like what diabetics use for insulin injections.

Biologics also come as infusions. To receive an infusion, you would go to an infusion center once every month or so. An IV is started, similar to when you get blood drawn. The medicine is given through the IV over an hour or so, and then the IV is taken out. An infusion nurse is there to monitor your vital signs and check for any side effects while you are receiving the infusion.

Do the newer treatments have more side effects?

The biologics don't have *more* side effects, but they have *different* side effects. Whereas DMARDs are processed though the liver and can affect the liver enzymes, the biologics have very little metabolism through the liver and are safe with liver and kidney dysfunction. They aren't pills that can cause stomach upset, nausea, or diarrhea, so they are a good choice for patients with sensitive stomachs.

The biologics tend to have black box warnings for increased risk of infections or atypical infections, since they do suppress the immune system. They can also have a black box warning for increased risk of lymphoma and malignancies.

Do biologics cause cancer?

It is unclear from research studies whether rheumatoid arthritis patients had a slightly increased risk of lymphoma to begin with, due to increased inflammation within their lymph nodes, or whether the slightly increased risk is actually due to the biologic medications themselves. In any case, the FDA required the black box warning to be placed on the labels of some of the biologics.

Rheumatologists typically avoid biologics such as Humira or Enbrel when a patient has an active or recent case of cancer. There are some biologics that are considered safe with a history of cancer, such as Orencia, which will be discussed in an upcoming section.

Do biologics cause tuberculosis?

Biologics don't cause tuberculosis, but if a patient already has latent tuberculosis before starting a biologic, the latent tuberculosis can become activated into full-blown tuberculosis. For this reason, rheumatologists check a tuberculosis test on every patient prior to starting a biologic, especially the TNF inhibitors.

The tuberculosis test is usually a blood test called a Quantiferon TB Gold. Some rheumatologists also perform a chest x-ray, depending on the patient's risk factors, such as recent travel to an endemic area.

What is the benefit of taking injectable or infusions over tablets?

When patients can't take DMARDs such as methotrexate due to stomach upset or elevated liver enzymes, the biologics become an attractive choice. The biologics don't cause stomach upset because they are injected under the skin rather than taken as a pill. They are not metabolized by the liver and do not affect the liver or kidneys, so they don't cause stress on the liver or kidneys in patients who already have these organ problems.

Injectable medications and infusions also stay in the body for longer periods of time, so they don't need to be taken every day. Injectables are usually taken once per week or every other week. Infusions can be given anywhere from once a month to once every six months, depending on which medication it is.

There is no alcohol restriction or eye exams required at regular intervals with biologics. There are no blood draws required every three months to monitor your labs with biologics.

How much will my immune system be suppressed with taking a biologic? Will I catch the cold and flu more easily than other people?

Biologic medications only suppress a portion of the immune system, not the entire apparatus. Your body will still be able to fight off infections, but it may take longer to recover from infections than others. Most of my patients taking biologics had very mild COVID infection symptoms and did not report an increased rate of infections overall.

Can biologics be taken together with a DMARD?

Yes, many patients are taking both a DMARD and a biologic together because they work synergistically. The benefit of taking a DMARD along with a biologic is that the DMARD actually increases biologic levels by 30% in the body. A biologic can build up to therapeutic levels much faster when a patient is taking a DMARD concurrently. For example, a lot of my patients continue to take methotrexate even after adding Humira therapy.

Sometimes the immune system can develop resistance to a biologic by producing antibodies against it after a period of time. DMARDs like methotrexate protect the body from producing antibodies against biologics. This means that the biologics can work better for a longer period of time without having to switch to another medication.

Since biologics are not processed by the liver, there is no additional stress on the liver from taking a DMARD and biologic together. Reasons to discontinue a DMARD after starting a biologic are stomach upset, liver enzyme elevation that has already occurred before starting the biologic, or any of the other side effects we discussed in the previous chapter.

Benefits of taking a DMARD with a biologic

Increase in biologic levels by 30% in the body
Prevention of antibody development against biologics
Synergistic effect with two medications together
Increased joint protection and symptom resolution

Can two biologics be combined together?

No, it is considered excessive immunosuppression to combine two or more biologics together. The benefit of combining biologics has not been proven, and the risk is too high for developing atypical infections and other side effects.

Are biologics safe during pregnancy and breastfeeding?

Biologics are usually avoided during pregnancy and breastfeeding. There aren't enough research studies done on biologics during pregnancy to say whether they are really safe or not. Since we don't know for sure how a biologic would affect a developing fetus in utero, they are not generally considered safe for use. We only use biologics during pregnancy when a mother is really suffering from her arthritis and she feels that the benefit would outweigh the potential risk.

The only biologic that is safe during pregnancy is one called Cimzia. Cimzia is special in that it is "pegylated," meaning it is attached to a molecule that prevents it from crossing the placental barrier entirely. The fetus and placenta are completely protected from Cimzia in the bloodstream and tissues. For that reason, a lot of my younger female patients who have plans to start a family are taking Cimzia.

Can I receive vaccines while taking a biologic?

Yes, you can receive any vaccine that is an inactivated vaccine—such as the flu shot, new shingles shot, and other inactive ones. Avoid live vaccines such as the flu nasal mist and the measles/mumps/rubella vaccine.

Will biologics blunt my immune system's response to vaccines?

There is some evidence that the immune system doesn't respond as well to vaccinations while under the influence of immunosuppressants. If you want to maximize and optimize your immune system's response to a vaccine—for example the COVID-19 vaccine—you could try stopping your biologic temporarily before receiving the vaccine, and then restart it later. Vaccines will be discussed more in chapter 9, "Navigating rheumatoid arthritis during the COVID-19 pandemic."

TNF INHIBITORS

What is "TNF"?

TNF stands for "tumor necrosis factor" and is a substance in the body produced by immune cells. TNF is highly inflammatory and triggers an inflammatory cascade to signal other cells to produce inflammation as well. Research has shown that TNF is a key player in the vicious cycle of rheumatoid arthritis.

Patients with rheumatoid arthritis often have TNF levels that are much higher than the general population. By blocking the TNF molecule in the body, a great deal of inflammation is reduced and patients feel significantly better with less joint pain and swelling.

What are TNF inhibitors?

TNF inhibitors are monoclonal antibodies or decoy receptors that directly block the TNF molecule or prevent it from reaching its destination on cells. The ultimate effect is that the TNF molecule cannot bind to its target receptor and isn't able to do what it typically does in producing inflammation and signaling other cells to produce inflammatory markers.

What are examples of TNF inhibitors?

- Humira (adalimumab)
- Enbrel (etanercept)
- Remicade (infliximab)
- Simponi (golimumab)
- Cimzia (certolizumab pegol)

Mechanism of Action

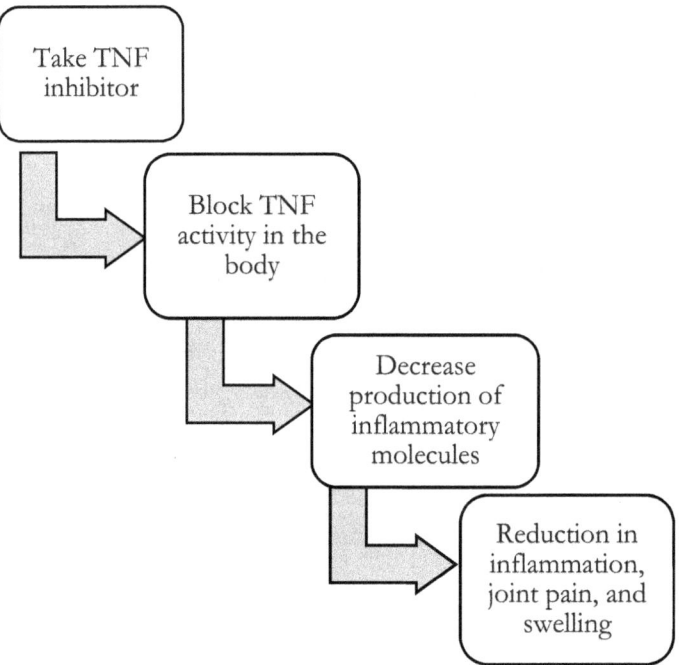

How are TNF inhibitors administered?

TNF inhibitors are taken as injections under the skin, rather than a pill by mouth. Needles can sound scary, but the injections are relatively easy to give. For a lot of these injectable medications, the needle is mostly hidden and is very small.

For example, Humira comes in an autoinjector pen that resembles an Epi-pen. Patients hold the pen against their skin, push a button, and the injection goes in over a few seconds. Sometimes the medication comes in a prefilled syringe (Cimzia) or a "cassette" that can be inserted into an injection device (Enbrel). For the most part, these medications have been designed to be user-friendly for patients who suffer from arthritis in their hand joints and may have reduced dexterity and mobility of their fingers.

The injection is usually given in the lower abdomen on the right or left side, or the upper thighs. The injection can also be given in the upper arms if there is a family member or friend with you who can help you. The frequency of the injections varies—please see the chart below.

Can TNF inhibitors also be given as infusions?

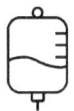

Yes, some of the TNF inhibitors have been formulated as infusions. Remicade (infliximab) is given as an infusion every 4-8 weeks. Simponi aria (golimumab) is given as an infusion every 4 weeks. Since infusions have better bioavailability in the body and last longer, they can be given with less frequency compared to the injections.

To receive an infusion, you would usually go to an infusion center at a hospital. A nurse would start an IV to give the medication over 1-2 hours, and then remove the IV after the infusion is completed.

Dosing Schedule of TNF inhibitors

Humira	1 injection every 2 weeks
Enbrel	1 injection every week
Remicade	1 infusion every 4-8 weeks
Simponi	1 injection every month
Simponi aria	1 infusion every month
Cimzia	1 injection every 2 weeks, or 2 injections every 4 weeks

How long does it take for TNF inhibitors to take effect?

It takes about 3 months on average for a TNF inhibitor to build up to therapeutic levels. Some patients say they feel a difference after the first injection, and some say it takes longer. Just like it is with the 3-month waiting period for DMARD medications, some patients may choose to take a temporary steroid taper while the biologic builds up to therapeutic levels.

What are the most common side effects of TNF inhibitors?

Patients have reported injection site reactions, such as redness, pain, or hives at the area of injection. To reduce injection site reactions, you can rotate between different injection sites and also apply ice to the area where you injected. Benadryl gel can also be applied on the injection site if there is itching or redness that develops.

What are rare side effects of TNF inhibitors?

In some cases, TNF inhibitors have contributed to development of opportunistic infections, which are infections that people with a normal immune system would not have gotten. These can include fungal or mycobacterial infections. For this reason, the FDA required a black box warning about increased risk of infections to be placed on the labels of TNF inhibitors.

Patients who are known to have stage 3-4 congestive heart failure, or demyelinating neurological conditions such as multiple sclerosis or Guillain-Barre syndrome should avoid taking a TNF inhibitor. Although TNF inhibitors don't <u>cause</u> these conditions, they can make underlying neurologic or congestive heart failure symptoms worse.

Do TNF inhibitors cause cancer?

In research studies, there was a slightly increased risk of lymphoma with use of TNF inhibitors. It was unclear from the studies whether the increased risk was due to underlying systemic inflammation from the disease process of rheumatoid arthritis itself, or whether the medications directly caused the increased risk.

In any case, the FDA required a black box warning to be placed about malignancies. Patients with active or recent malignancies should avoid TNF inhibitors.

Potential side effects of TNF inhibitors

Injection site reactions
Allergic reaction
Black box warning for lymphoma and malignancies
Black box warning for opportunistic infections
Worsening of stage 3-4 congestive heart failure
Worsening of demyelinating neurologic conditions

Do TNF inhibitors require routine bloodwork to be done?

There are no strict guidelines about doing routine bloodwork while a patient is taking a TNF inhibitor. Since TNF inhibitors don't affect the blood cell counts, kidneys, or liver to a significant extent, there is no requirement for lab work like there is with the DMARD medications.

Based on expert opinion, it's a good idea to get your labs checked about once per year while taking a TNF inhibitor, similar to what a primary care doctor would do for an annual physical.

Is there any reason I should avoid starting a TNF inhibitor?

Patients should avoid starting a TNF inhibitor for the following reasons:

- Any active infection that is still being treated with antibiotics or antimicrobials.
- Latent or active tuberculosis.

- Any history of active or recent cancer, especially lymphoma.
- Stage 3-4 congestive heart failure.
- History of multiple sclerosis, Guillain-Barre syndrome, or other demyelinating neurologic conditions.

Can my body develop resistance to a TNF inhibitor over time?

Sometimes patients report that their TNF inhibitor medication used to work really well, and it doesn't work as well anymore because they notice joint pain and swelling coming back. They can notice more hives at the injection site or other side effects developing over time. This can sometimes indicate that the body has developed resistance against the TNF inhibitor.

For example, since Humira is a monoclonal antibody, the body can actually recognize it as a foreign molecule and develop antibodies against it. This typically happens if a patient has been taking a biologic for a long time and then stops taking it for some reason (an illness, surgery, or sometimes life circumstances or insurance issues). When the biologic is restarted, the body now sees it as a foreign substance and has developed resistance against it.

If your rheumatologist suspects that this has happened, he or she might check special labs to see if your body produced antibodies against the medication. The labs could help decide whether to continue the same medication or switch to a new one.

Summary of TNF inhibitors:

- TNF inhibitors were the first class of biologics ever developed.
- They target a highly inflammatory molecule in the body known to contribute to rheumatoid arthritis symptoms and progression.
- They are very effective at reducing joint pain, swelling, stiffness, and protecting the joints against damage and deformity.
- They come as injectables and infusions.
- Avoid them with active infections, congestive heart failure stage 3-4, a history of demyelinating neurologic conditions such as multiple sclerosis and Guillain Barre syndrome, and active or previous history of malignancy and lymphoma.
- The only TNF inhibitor that is safe in pregnancy is Cimzia, which cannot cross the placental barrier.

IL-6 INHIBITORS

What is "IL-6"?

IL-6 stands for "interleukin 6" and is a substance in the body produced by immune cells. IL-6 is a highly inflammatory cytokine and triggers an inflammatory cascade to signal other cells to produce inflammation as well. Research has shown that IL-6 is another key player in the vicious cycle of rheumatoid arthritis.

Patients with rheumatoid arthritis often have IL-6 levels that are much higher compared to the general population. By blocking the IL-6 molecule in the body, a great deal of inflammation is reduced and patients feel significantly better with less joint pain and swelling.

What are IL-6 inhibitors?

IL-6 inhibitors are monoclonal antibodies that directly block the IL-6 molecule or prevent it from reaching its destination on cells. The ultimate effect is that the IL-6 cytokine cannot bind to its target receptor and isn't able to do what it typically does in producing inflammation and signaling other cells to produce inflammatory markers.

What are the two IL-6 inhibitors?

- Actemra (tocilizumab)
- Kevzara (sarilumab)

How are IL-6 inhibitors administered?

IL-6 inhibitors are also taken as injections under the skin. The injections usually come as a prefilled syringe or a pen.

The injection is usually given in the lower abdomen on the right or left side, or the upper thighs. The injection can also be given in the upper arms if there is a family member or friend with you who can help you.

Can IL-6 inhibitors also be given as infusions?

Yes, Actemra (tocilizumab) can be given as an infusion. Since infusions have better bioavailability in the body and last longer, they can be given with less frequency compared to the injections.

Mechanism of Action

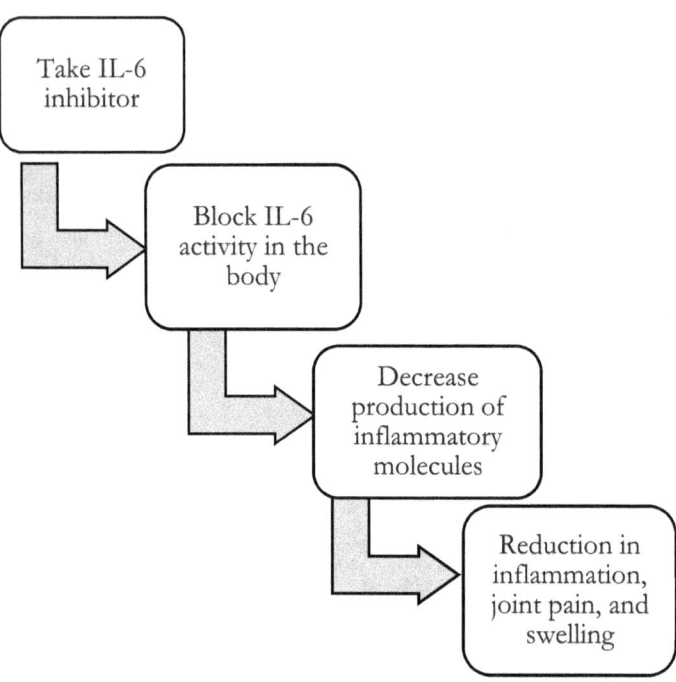

Dosing Schedule of IL-6 inhibitors

Actemra	1 injection every week or 1 infusion every month
Kevzara	1 injection every 2 weeks

How long does it take for IL-6 inhibitors to take effect?

It takes about 3 months on average for an IL-6 inhibitor to build up to therapeutic levels. Some patients say they feel a difference after the first injection, and some say it takes longer.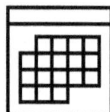

What are the most common side effects of IL-6 inhibitors?

Patients have reported injection site reactions, such as redness, pain, or hives at the area of injection. To reduce injection site reactions, you can rotate between different injection sites and also apply ice to the area where you injected. Benadryl gel can also be applied on the injection site if there is itching or redness that develops.

What are rare side effects of IL-6 inhibitors?

Research studies found an increased risk in bowel perforations, especially in patients with previously known diverticulitis. Patients who have diverticulitis or a history of bowel perforation should avoid IL-6 inhibitors.

IL-6 inhibitors, especially Actemra, can also worsen elevated liver enzymes. Actemra is usually avoided when liver enzymes are already elevated.

Do IL-6 inhibitors cause cancer?

Research studies did not show a significant increase in lymphoma or other malignancies with the use of IL-6 inhibitors.

Do IL-6 inhibitors require routine bloodwork to be done?

Labs should be done prior to starting an IL-6 inhibitor to make sure liver enzymes are normal. Blood work is then checked every 6 months to 1 year to keep an eye on the liver enzymes.

Is there any reason I should avoid taking an IL-6 inhibitor?

Patients should avoid starting an IL-6 inhibitor for the following reasons:

- Any active infection that is still being treated.
- Elevated liver enzymes.
- Diverticulitis or history of bowel perforation.
- Inflammatory bowel disease such as Crohn's disease or ulcerative colitis which poses a risk of bowel perforation.

Research studies have <u>not</u> shown an increase in the risk of malignancies, worsening of congestive heart failure, or worsening of demyelinating neurological conditions such as multiple sclerosis.

Potential side effects of IL-6 inhibitors

Injection site reactions
Allergic reaction
Elevated liver enzymes
Bowel perforation (avoid with diverticulitis)
Black box warning for opportunistic infections
High cholesterol levels

Summary of IL-6 inhibitors:

- IL-6 inhibitors include Actemra and Kevzara.
- They are usually used as second or third-line biologics if the TNF inhibitors don't work or should be avoided.
- They come as injections and infusions.
- They are typically not associated with an increase in lymphoma or cancers, but they are associated with risk of bowel perforation in patients with diverticulitis or other bowel conditions predisposing to perforation.
- They can be used alone or together with a DMARD medication. Two biologics cannot be combined together.

B-CELL and T-CELL INHIBITORS

What are B-cells?

B-cells are involved in the immune system's long-term memory. They produce molecules called antibodies that can remember which viruses and bacteria the body has been exposed to in the past, and can mount a quick response if the same exposure occurs again.

In autoimmune diseases, B-cells also produce the auto-antibodies that are aimed against the body's own tissues. This includes rheumatoid factor and the anti-CCP antibodies that were mentioned previously. These antibodies lead to inflammation that result in joint pain and damage over time.

What are T-cells?

T-cells come in two types, helper T-cells and killer T-cells. As the name suggests, helper T-cells enable other cells in the body to become activated by sending them signals to attack a foreign bacteria or virus. Also appropriately named, killer T-cells are the assassins that take out the bacteria and viruses that are foreign invaders in our body.

In autoimmune diseases, T-cells attack our own body tissues rather than foreign bacteria or viruses. They also release signals (called cytokines) to start a cascade of inflammation to activate other cells to carry out similar tasks.

What are B-cell and T-cell inhibitors?

B and T-cell inhibitors are medications that stop these cells from producing the inflammation and damage to joints that usually occur once an autoimmune disease has been triggered. These medications are biologics that block certain pathways in the activation of B and T-cells.

What are examples of B-cell and T-cell inhibitors?

- Orencia (abatacept)
- Rituxan (rituximab)

How does Orencia (abatacept) work?

Orencia blocks a pathway called "co-stimulation" of T-cells. T-cells usually require two signals to become fully activated, otherwise they become inactivated and fade away without the second signal. By blocking this second signal, Orencia decreases the activation of T-cells and reduces their attack on joint tissues.

Mechanism of Action

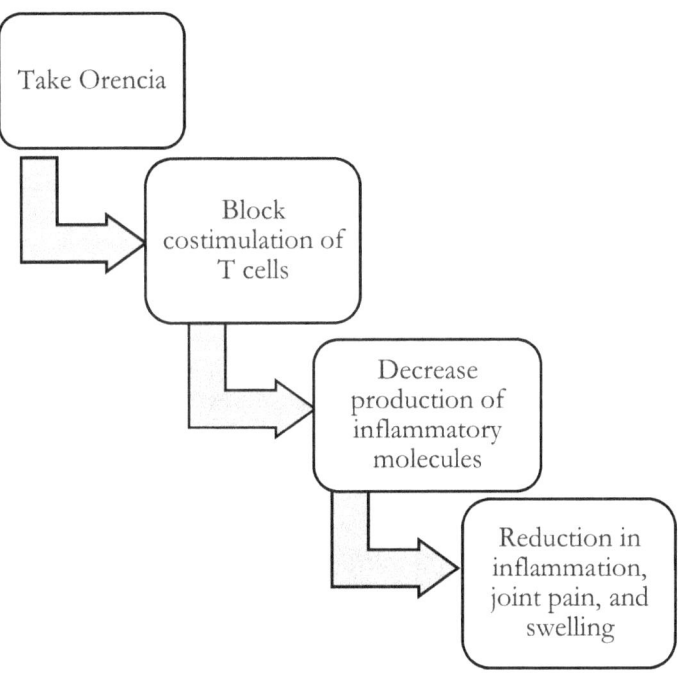

How is Orencia administered?

Orencia is given as a 125 mg injection under the skin once per week at home. Orencia also comes as an infusion that can be given every 4 weeks at an infusion center.

What are the most common side effects of Orencia?

Orencia can cause injection site reaction, such as redness, itching, hives, or bruising. If Orencia is given as an infusion, it can also cause infusion reactions with symptoms similar to an allergic reaction, such as a rash.

Potential side effects of Orencia

Injection site reactions
Infusion reactions
Headaches

Does Orencia cause cancer?

No, Orencia is one of the biologics that have not been shown to have an increased risk of cancer, including lymphoma, in research studies. It is also not shown to be associated with an increased risk of tuberculosis or atypical infections.

Does Orencia require routine bloodwork to be done?

There are no set guidelines for the frequency of bloodwork while receiving Orencia. Expert opinions say that annual labs once per year are prudent in patients taking biologics.

Is there any reason I should avoid taking Orencia?

Patients should not start Orencia if they have any active or serious infection that has not completed treatment.

How does Rituxan (rituximab) work?

Rituximab works by blocking the activity of B-cells, the ones that produce antibodies. By blocking a receptor called

"CD20" on B-cells, they no longer receive a signal to proliferate in the bloodstream.

Mechanism of Action

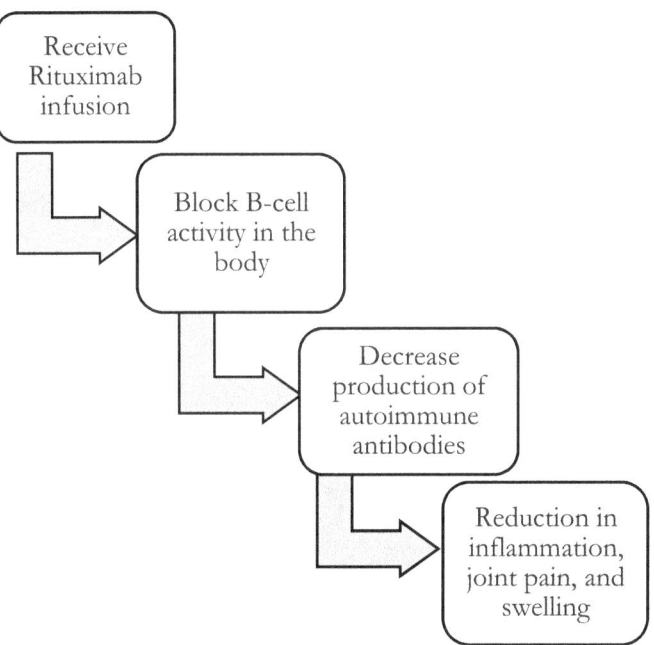

How is rituximab administered?

Rituximab only comes as an infusion, given intravenously at an infusion center. Rituximab is usually given as 2 doses every 6 months. There is currently no injectable form of rituximab that can be given at home.

Rituximab also comes in "biosimilar" versions, which means that there are generic forms of the original medication that are less costly but work just as effectively and have the same drug safety and side effect profile.

What are the most common side effects of rituximab?

Rituximab can cause infusion reactions, such as rashes, low blood pressure, or symptoms similar to an allergic reaction. There is also an increased risk of opportunistic infections while receiving rituximab. The infusion can result in low blood cell counts or neutropenia (low white blood cells that fight infection).

Pre-medications are usually given with each rituximab infusion. These usually include Tylenol, Benadryl, and an IV steroid given right before the infusion to prevent side effects such as allergic reactions from occurring.

Potential side effects of rituximab

Infusion reaction or allergic reaction
Low blood cell counts or neutropenia
Opportunistic infections

Does rituximab cause cancer?

No, there is no increased risk of cancer with use of rituximab. In fact, rituximab is actually used in certain chemotherapy regimens for treatment of lymphoma. This makes rituximab a suitable choice in patients who have active cancer or lymphoma in addition to severe rheumatoid arthritis symptoms.

Does rituximab require routine bloodwork to be done?

Yes, blood cell counts need to be monitored with each rituximab infusion since it can lower blood cell counts unexpectedly.

Is there any reason I should avoid taking rituximab?

Patients should not start rituximab if they have any active or serious infection, or if they have low blood cell counts to begin with.

Summary of B and T cell inhibitors:

- Orencia and Rituximab both block the function of overactive B and T cells in autoimmune disease.
- These biologics do not have an increased risk of malignancy or lymphoma.
- They come as injectables or infusions.
- Orencia may be the safest biologic for patients with a history of malignancy or those who are at high risk for opportunistic infections such as tuberculosis.

SUMMARY OF BIOLOGIC TREATMENTS

	Injectable	Infusion	Black box warning for malignancy	Black box warning for infections	Avoid with congestive heart failure	Avoid with demyelinating neurologic conditions (multiple sclerosis, GBS)	Safe in pregnancy and breastfeeding	Requires routine blood monitoring
Humira	✓		✓	✓	✓	✓		
Enbrel	✓		✓	✓	✓	✓		
Remicade		✓	✓	✓	✓	✓		
Simponi	✓	✓	✓	✓	✓	✓		
Cimzia	✓		✓	✓	✓	✓	✓	
Actemra	✓	✓		✓				✓
Kevzara	✓			✓				
Orencia	✓	✓						
Rituximab	✓	✓		✓				✓

Final Thoughts on Biologics

Should I skip a dose of my biologic medication if I'm sick with a cold or fever?

If you are sick, the rule is that you should pause your biologic if you have a fever or require antibiotics for any infection. After your fever has resolved and/or the antibiotics are completed, you can restart the biologic.

Do I have to take a biologic forever? When do I stop taking this medication?

Typically, patients do take a biologic long-term. If the biologic keeps working and there are no side effects, we typically don't stop the medication or flares of rheumatoid arthritis will occur.

However, if the body develops resistance against the biologic or if you are experiencing side effects such as injection site reactions, you could discuss with your rheumatologist discontinuing the medication or switching to another one.

Do biologics have to stay refrigerated?

Yes, these medications have to stay cold and are usually stored in the fridge until you are ready to use it. If the medication stays in room temperature for too long, it becomes inactivated. Do not freeze a biologic medication.

If you are traveling overseas with a biologic, you have to carry it with you in a cold case on the airplane until you can get to your hotel and put it in the mini fridge.

Financial and Insurance Considerations

How well does insurance cover biologics? Are these medications expensive?

Biologics are usually very expensive before insurance pays its portion. For example, Humira costs around $3,000 per month before insurance coverage. Insurance usually requires that one DMARD, usually methotrexate, be tried before switching to a biologic. For patients with commercial insurance, there is good coverage of biologic medications. Commercially insured patients can use a copay card which will bring down the cost to $0 or $5 per month after insurance pays their portion.

Things get a bit trickier with Medicare and government-sponsored types of insurance. Patients can fall into the "Medicare donut hole," which means that Medicare covers the biologic cost up to a certain amount, but then the patient has to pay the rest on their own until they reach a certain limit ("catastrophic coverage"). This can be a very difficult situation since the cost of biologics can be thousands of dollars per month while a patient is in the donut hole.

Fortunately, there are patient assistance programs offered by the drug companies. Patients can apply for these assistance programs, and if their household income qualifies, they can usually receive the biologic medication for free.

Some Medicare plans cover infusions better than injectable medications at home, since infusions are usually billed under Medicare Part B (hospital and medical coverage), whereas home injections are usually covered under Medicare Part D (prescription and drug coverage). Check with your rheumatologist whether your insurance plan might cover infusions better than injectable medications if the cost of biologics becomes a barrier for you.

Case scenarios

These case scenarios are illustrations of journeys that different patients may experience, which are loosely based on the paths that some of my patients have taken with biologic medications. Names have been changed for anonymity.

Case 1

After increasing her dose of methotrexate to maximum levels, Sharon is quite frustrated that she only feels 50-70% better from her rheumatoid arthritis symptoms. She talked to her rheumatologist about what to do next, and together they decided to add Humira, which is one injection every other week.

Sharon finds that the Humira injections are quite easy to give and the autoinjector pen that the medicine comes in is really user friendly for her arthritic hands and sting-free. They decided to continue the methotrexate along with the Humira because they work together synergistically. Within 1-2 months of starting Humira, Sharon feels a lot better and isn't reporting any side effects from her medications at follow up appointments.

Case 2

Mary has rheumatoid arthritis and usually takes methotrexate, which has worked well for years. However, she just got married and wants to start a family soon. She's wondering what medications she could take that would be safe for pregnancy and breastfeeding.

She and her rheumatologist discuss that she will have to stop methotrexate before attempting to conceive because it's not safe for a developing fetus. They decide to start Cimzia injections instead, since this is the only biologic that is considered safe in pregnancy.

Case 3

Keith was recently diagnosed with prostate cancer which has metastasized to the liver. He received chemotherapy and radiation and is currently considered stable with his prostate cancer. Unfortunately, it has been a rough year and Keith started experiencing joint pain and swelling as well. He was diagnosed with rheumatoid arthritis and is wondering what treatments would be safe with his history of prostate cancer.

To avoid additional stress on the liver, his rheumatologist decided to avoid DMARD medications. They discussed Orencia, the biologic considered to be the safest in patients with a history of cancer. Keith starts giving himself one injection per week at home and feels that the injection device is easy to give. He starts feeling better in about 1-2 months.

Reflection questions:

1. What aspects of biologic treatments seem like they would be a good fit with you?

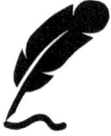

2. What aspects of biologic treatments seem concerning to you?

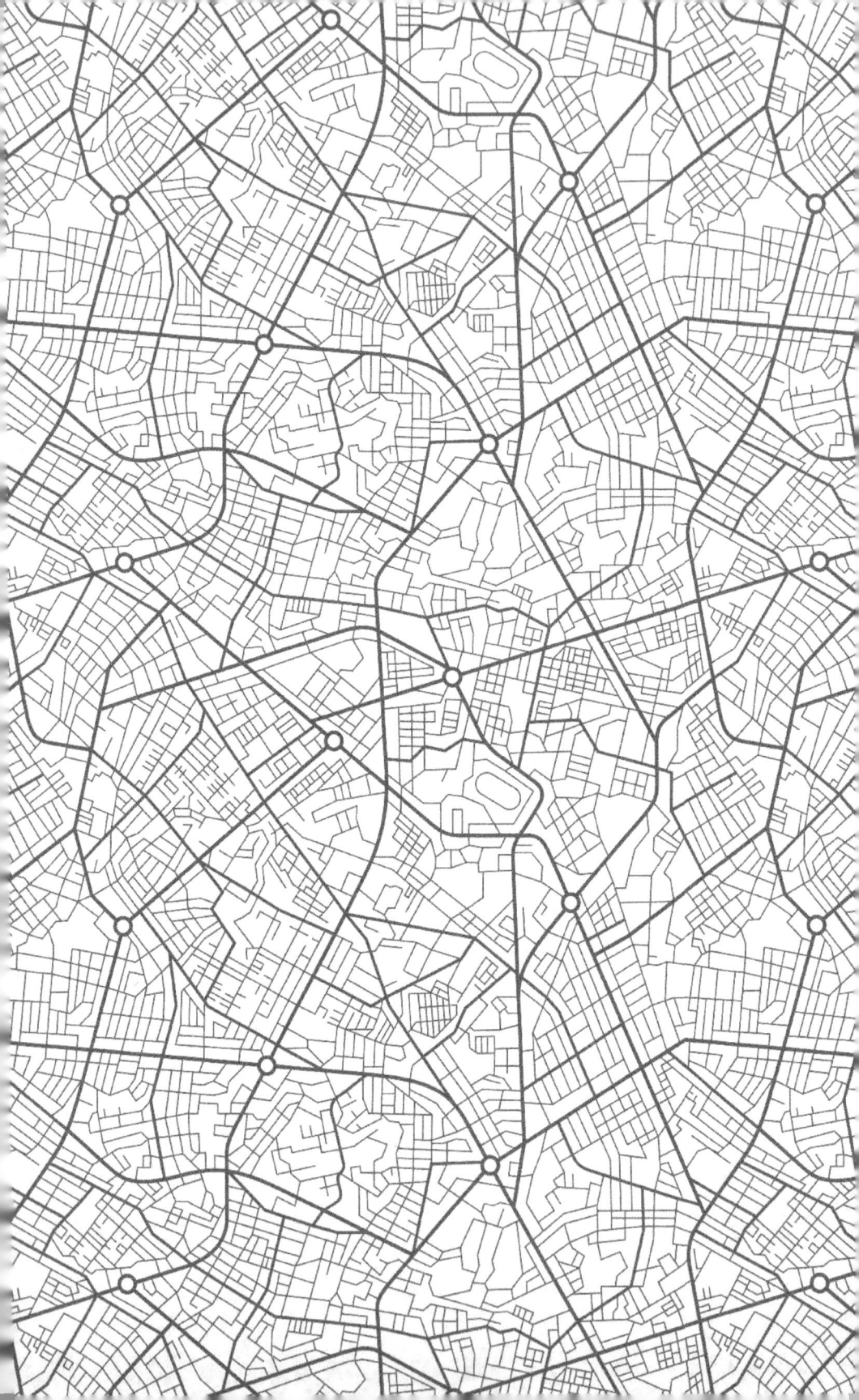

CHAPTER 5
NAVIGATING THE JAK INHIBITORS

BREAKTHROUGHS IN RHEUMATOID ARTHRITIS TREATMENT

What is "JAK"?

Pronounced just like "Jack"—as in Jack and Jill—the JAK receptor is short for "janus kinase." Named after Janus, the two-faced god in Greek mythology, the janus kinase receptor is located on the border of cells and is responsible for multiple signaling pathways involved in activating immune cells and producing inflammation in the body.

There are multiple JAK receptors, known as JAK1, JAK2, JAK3, and TYK2. When a JAK receptor is activated, it triggers increased production of inflammatory markers to be made downstream by activating DNA transcription. In other words, there is increased genetic expression of inflammatory end-products.

What are JAK inhibitors?

JAK inhibitors are a relatively new class of medications. These are not biologics, but rather called "small molecules." Instead of blocking targeting one molecule, such as TNF or IL-6, they block the JAK receptor that is responsible for producing a multitude of inflammatory molecules.

Due to blocking so many inflammatory markers at once, the JAK inhibitors tend to work faster, within 2 weeks or so, in contrast to DMARDS and biologics which take about 2-3 months to build up to therapeutic levels.

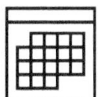

What was the first JAK inhibitor that was developed?

Xeljanz, also known as tofacitinib, is the first known JAK inhibitor, and it was developed by Pfizer. Xeljanz was approved by the FDA in use for patients with rheumatoid arthritis in 2012. This is a new and exciting era for rheumatoid arthritis since a new mechanism of action was found to treat this painful condition. Rheumatoid arthritis patients need more options for therapy in case older medications don't work or cause side effects. Many new JAK inhibitors have been developed and several are undergoing research trials for FDA approval.

How many JAK inhibitors are available now for rheumatoid arthritis?

- Xeljanz (tofacitinib)
- Rinvoq (upadacitinib)
- Olumiant (baricitinib)
- Brepocitinib—still under research and development
- Filgotinib—still under research and development

How is a JAK inhibitor taken?

JAK inhibitors come as tablets that are taken on a daily basis. They are not available as injectables or infusions.

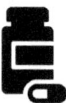

Dosing schedule of JAK inhibitors

Xeljanz 5 mg twice daily or 11 mg once daily
Rinvoq 15 mg once daily
Olumiant 2 mg once daily

Mechanism of Action

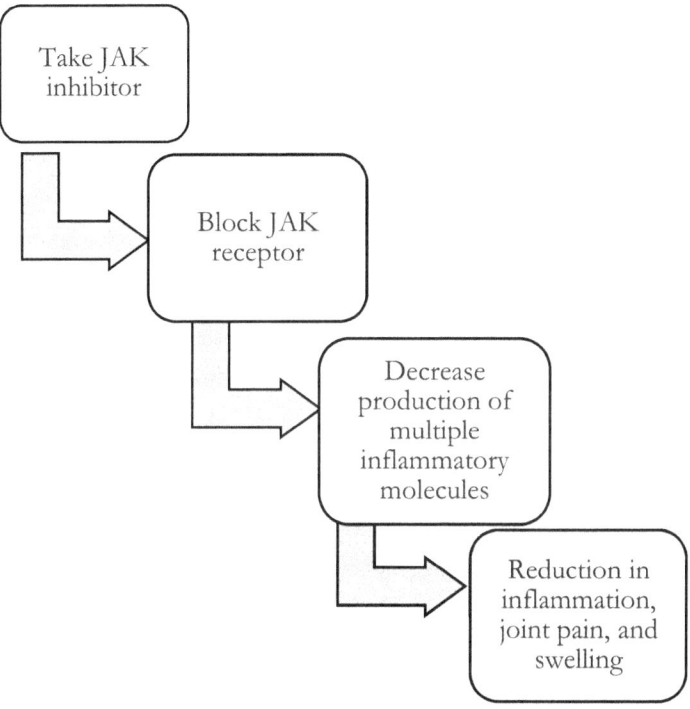

What are potential side effects of the JAK inhibitors?

Any medication taken as a pill can cause stomach upset or nausea. However, there are less digestive side effects reported with JAK inhibitors compared with DMARDs such as methotrexate.

JAK inhibitors have a few black box warnings. Similar to biologics, there is a warning for increased risk of infections, as well as increased risk of lymphoma and malignancies.

Another warning is for increased risk of cardiovascular disease such as heart attacks and strokes. However, in the studies that showed this risk, it was mainly the group of patients who were over age 65 with traditional risk factors for heart disease, such as obesity, diabetes, high blood pressure, smoking, and high cholesterol, that developed issues.

Potential side effects of JAK inhibitors

Nausea, vomiting, stomach pain
Elevated liver enzymes
Soft stools or diarrhea
Elevated cholesterol levels
Increased risk of DVT (blood clots)
Black box warning for cardiovascular events such as heart attack or stroke
Black box warning for opportunistic infections
Black box warning for lymphoma and malignancies

Do JAK inhibitors cause cancer?

In research studies, there was a slightly increased risk of lymphoma with use of JAK inhibitors. It was unclear from the studies whether the increased risk was due to underlying systemic inflammation from the disease process of rheumatoid arthritis itself, or whether the medications directly caused the increased risk.

In any case, the FDA required a black box warning to be placed about malignancies. Patients with active or recent malignancies should avoid JAK inhibitors.

Do JAK inhibitors cause tuberculosis?

JAK inhibitors don't cause tuberculosis, but if a patient already has latent tuberculosis before starting it, the latent tuberculosis can become activated into full-blown tuberculosis. For this reason, rheumatologists check a tuberculosis test on every patient prior to starting a JAK inhibitor.

The tuberculosis test is usually a blood test called a Quantiferon TB Gold. Some rheumatologists also perform a chest x-ray, depending on the patient's risk factors, such as recent travel to an endemic area.

Can JAK inhibitors help with the fatigue component of rheumatoid arthritis?

Yes, Xeljanz was specifically studied for fatigue in patients with rheumatoid arthritis. According to the study, patients not only experienced improvement in joint pain and function, but they also experienced an improvement in their fatigue and energy levels.

The improvement in fatigue may be due to decreased systemic inflammation from treatment, or an increase in sleep quality after resolution of joint pain and discomfort at night. Other JAK inhibitors are also being studied for the same effect on fatigue.

Can JAK inhibitors be taken together with a DMARD?

Yes, many patients are taking both a DMARD and a JAK inhibitor together because they work synergistically. For example, methotrexate and Xeljanz can be taken together, and are taken together quite frequently.

There is a bit more increased stress on the liver because both medications are processed by the liver. Your rheumatologist will keep a close eye on lab monitoring every 3 months.

Can JAK inhibitors be taken together with a biologic?

No, it is considered excessive immunosuppression to combine JAK inhibitors and biologics together. The benefit of combining them has not been proven, and the risk is too high for developing atypical infections and having other side effects.

Are JAK inhibitors safe during pregnancy and breastfeeding?

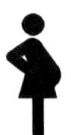

JAK inhibitors are usually avoided during pregnancy and breastfeeding. There aren't enough research studies done on these newer medications during pregnancy to say whether they are really safe or not. Since we don't know for sure how a Jak inhibitor would affect a developing fetus in utero, they are not generally considered safe for use. Avoid these medications during breastfeeding as well.

Do JAK inhibitors require routine lab monitoring and blood work to be done?

Yes, JAK inhibitors can cause liver enzyme elevations. They can also worsen your cholesterol levels. Your rheumatologist will typically get blood work done every 3 months to make sure everything is okay. Your rheumatologist may check your lipid panel prior to starting the medication, and then every 6 months or once per year to make sure your cholesterol isn't getting too high.

Can I receive vaccines while taking a JAK inhibitor?

Yes, you can receive any vaccine that is an <u>inactivated</u> vaccine—such as the flu shot, new shingles shot, and other inactive ones. Avoid <u>live vaccines</u> such as the flu nasal mist and the measles/mumps/rubella vaccine.

Will JAK inhibitors blunt my immune system's response to vaccines?

There is evidence that the immune system doesn't respond as well to vaccinations while under the influence of immunosuppressants. If you want to maximize and optimize your immune system's response to a vaccine—for example the COVID-19 vaccine—you could try stopping your immunosuppressant medication temporarily before receiving the vaccine, and then restart it later.

Financial and Insurance Considerations

How well does insurance cover JAK inhibitors? Are these medications expensive?

JAK inhibitors are usually very expensive before insurance pays its portion. As an example, Xeljanz costs about $5,000 per month before insurance coverage. Just like with biologics, insurance usually requires that one DMARD, usually methotrexate, be tried before adding or switching to a JAK inhibitor.

For patients with commercial insurance, there is good coverage of JAK inhibitors. Commercially insured patients can use a copay card which will bring down the cost to $0 or $5 per month after insurance pays their portion.

Things get a bit trickier with Medicare and government sponsored types of insurance. Patients can fall into the "Medicare donut hole," which means that Medicare covers the medication cost up to a certain amount, and then the patient has to pay the rest on their own until they reach a certain limit ("catastrophic coverage"). This can be very difficult since the cost of these medications can be thousands of dollars per month while a patient is in the donut hole.

Fortunately, there are options such as patient assistance programs offered by the drug companies. Patients can apply for these assistance programs, and if their household income qualifies, they can usually receive the medication for free.

Case scenarios

These case scenarios are illustrations of journeys that different patients may experience, which are loosely based on the paths that some of my patients have taken with the JAK inhibitors. Names have been changed for anonymity.

Case 1

Albert has tried all the DMARD medications since his rheumatoid arthritis diagnosis one year ago. He has a really sensitive stomach and he experienced a lot of stomach upset and diarrhea with all of the pills he tried so far. He is scared of needles and wants to avoid injectable biologic medications.

He saw a television commercial about Xeljanz and wants to give it a try. He starts the medication and feels like it starts working faster than the other medications he has tried up to now. He doesn't experience any stomach upset with Xeljanz and gets his labs checked every 3 months which remain stable.

Case 2

Gloria took Xeljanz for about two months and didn't feel like it was particularly helpful. She didn't have any side effects, but she didn't feel relief of her joint pain and swelling. Her rheumatologist suggested trying a different JAK inhibitor called Rinvoq instead. Gloria wonders how much different this other medication could be if it's from the same family of medications, and whether or not it would work on her.

Her rheumatologist explains that some patients can respond to one JAK inhibitor even if they have not responded to another one, and this is for unclear reasons. Gloria decides to go ahead and give Rinvoq a try, and it starts working within two weeks of starting it. She gets her labs drawn every 3 months and they remain normal. She doesn't have side effects to Rinvoq and continues taking it long-term.

Case 3

Jim has been taking a JAK inhibitor for about two years and it has always worked really well for him. However, on his most recent lab work, his cholesterol levels increased quite a bit. His cardiologist is really concerned because Jim has a family history of heart disease, and Jim has worsening cholesterol despite taking cholesterol medication.

Jim and his rheumatologist discuss whether to stay on his JAK inhibitor, which Jim is hesitant to give up because it works so well for his rheumatoid arthritis, or whether to switch to a different therapy. After thinking about it for a while, Jim decides he will try a different medication to see if it could just as well.

Reflection questions:

1. What aspects of JAK inhibitor treatments seem like they would be a good fit with you?

2. What aspects of JAK inhibitor treatments seem concerning to you?

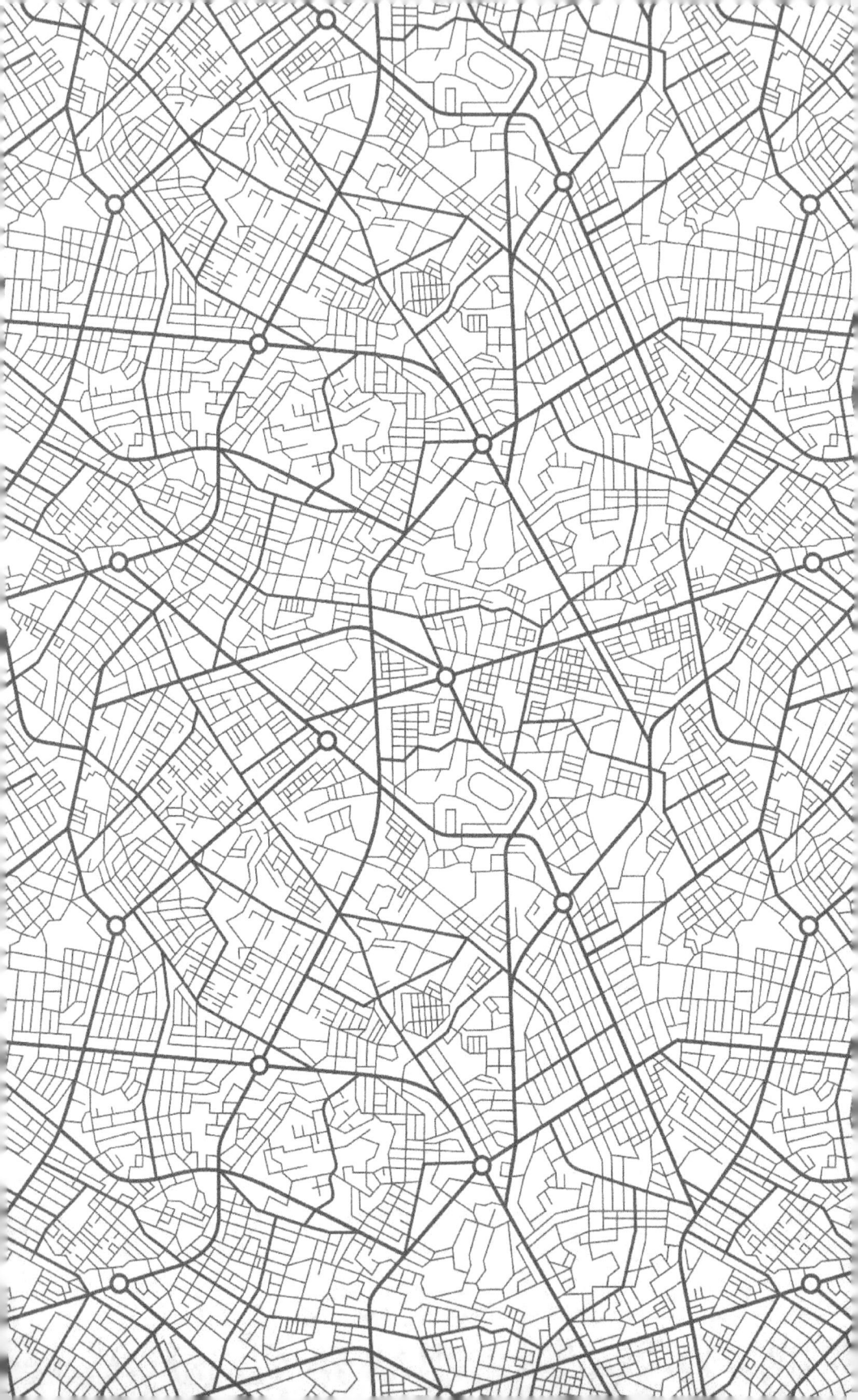

CHAPTER 6

NAVIGATING STEROIDS AND OVER-THE-COUNTER MEDICATIONS

STEROIDS

What are steroids and how do they work?

Steroids are also known as glucocorticoids or corticosteroids, and they exert anti-inflammatory effects through multiple pathways in the body. They enter the nucleus of cells and prevent expression of pro-inflammatory genes on DNA, and they also inhibit production of inflammatory proteins from cells.

Our body produces its own form of steroid, called cortisol, from the adrenal glands. Cortisol is released on a rhythmic cycle during day-to-day living. It is released in higher levels during periods of increased stress or illness.

Steroids used in rheumatoid arthritis

Prednisone tablets
Prednisolone tablets (Medrol Dosepak)
IV forms of steroids such as Solu-Medrol
Injectable forms of steroids such as Depo-Medrol

What is the role of using steroids for rheumatoid arthritis?

Steroids can be used initially when a patient has a new diagnosis of rheumatoid arthritis and is trying to get their symptoms and pain under control. As we discussed previously, it can take 2-3 months for DMARDs and biologics to start working. This is an excruciatingly long period of time to wait with severe joint pain, swelling, and inability to function! Steroids can help during this initial period of time while a patient is waiting for long-term medications to kick in.

Steroids can also be helpful when a patient is experiencing a flare of their arthritis. Flares can occur with weather and barometric changes, stress, illness, and other factors. Taking a prednisone taper for a short period of time can help with getting through an arthritic flare faster.

Mechanism of Action

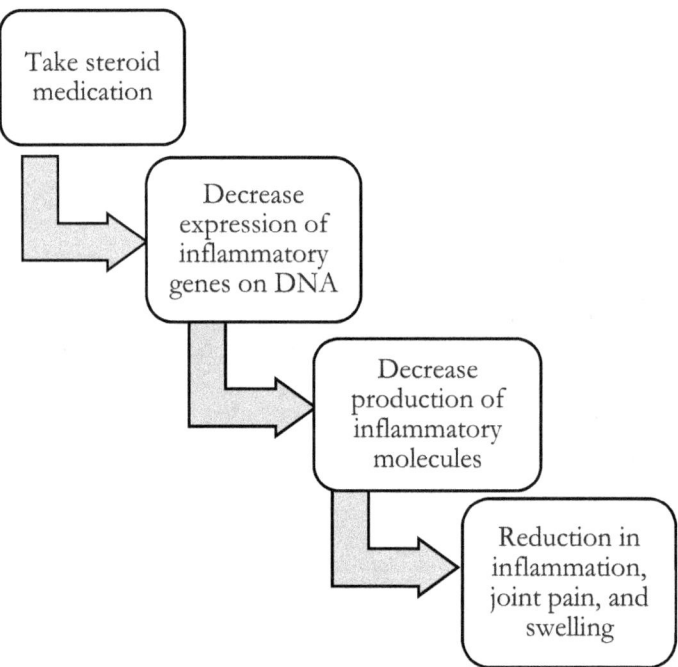

Why do steroids have to be tapered?

Since steroid tablets suppress our own adrenal glands' production of the cortisol hormone, stopping a steroid too suddenly could cause some unpleasant symptoms, like feeling weak, lightheaded, tired, or sick in general. The longer a patient has been on a steroid, the more dramatic this effect will be. It is a better idea to taper down slowly on a steroid in order to give the body a chance to catch up.

Is it okay to take a steroid long-term?

Taking a steroid medication for long periods of time, such as for months or years, is generally discouraged. Steroids are okay to take for a short period of time, but they have a lot of side effects when taken long-term, which we will review next.

Some patients report that they're unable to stop a steroid completely. They are stuck on low or medium doses of prednisone for a long time and feel really terrible if they try to wean down or discontinue. In that case, it's important to weigh the risks and benefits of taking a steroid for long periods of time with your rheumatologist.

Optimally, quality of life is maintained while side effects of medications are reduced as much as possible. The balance of risk versus quality of life will be different for each patient.

Can steroids worsen my blood sugar or cause diabetes?

Yes, steroids can worsen blood glucose and we try to avoid giving them at high doses in diabetic patients for that reason. If you don't have diabetes to begin with, your risk of developing it can increase with time as you continue to take a steroid.

Can steroids cause weight gain and increased appetite?

Yes, weight gain is one of the most common side effects reported with prednisone. Patients say that they gain a lot of weight with prednisone and can't get the weight off. They feel really hungry and "could eat everything in sight."

Can steroids disturb my mood and sleep patterns?

Yes, since steroids can change the body's natural production of the cortisol hormone, it can change your mood and sleep patterns. Patients report feeling more anxious or crabby while taking prednisone. They also report increased levels of energy during the day and insomnia at night.

Steroids like prednisone should be taken in the morning, as early as possible. Our body's natural release of cortisol is usually around 4:00 am in the morning before most of us are even out of bed. Prednisone should be taken with breakfast or first thing when you wake up. Avoid taking prednisone at night because it will contribute to insomnia and changes in circadian rhythm.

Can steroids cause skin changes like easy bruising and skin tearing?

Yes, steroids cause skin thinning and increases the fragility of skin. This can cause easy bruising, scratch marks that bleed easily, and prolonged wound healing time.

Can steroids cause "moon facies"?

Yes, steroids can make you gain weight in unexpected places like your face, and redistribute fat in your body to unpleasant places, such as the abdomen. "Moon facies" refers to a round appearance of the face in patients who take prednisone for long periods of time, either because they have to or because they're unable to wean off.

What is Cushing syndrome?

Cushing syndrome is the result of derangements in hormone levels in the body. A person taking steroids like prednisone for long periods of time can developing Cushing syndrome due to altered hormone levels. Symptoms of Cushing syndrome are weight gain, moon facies, wide stretch marks, fragile skin that bruises easily, acne, more body hair, fatigue, and other symptoms.

What is adrenal insufficiency in the context of steroids?

Adrenal insufficiency occurs when the body no longer produces enough of its own cortisol hormone because a patient has been taking steroid tablets for long periods of time. Prednisone suppresses the adrenal glands from producing its own natural form of steroids. Symptoms of adrenal insufficiency include fatigue, low blood pressure, weakness, low exercise tolerance, dizziness, and dehydration.

Can steroids cause fluid retention and swelling?

Yes, steroids can increase sodium and fluid retention. Patients have noticed increased swelling in the ankles and feet. Long-term steroids can be harmful in patients who have congestive heart failure or high blood pressure due to increased fluid and salt retention.

Can steroids cause osteoporosis?

Taking steroids for long periods of time can definitely increase your risk of osteoporosis. Steroids can weaken the bones and increase the future risk of a bone fracture. They also weaken muscles over time and cause loss of muscle mass.

Can steroids affect my eyes?

There is an increased risk of glaucoma and cataract formation in patients who take steroids long-term. Elevated blood sugar from steroids can also affect the eyes.

What is one of the most serious side effects of steroids?

Avascular necrosis is one of the most feared complications of steroids. This usually occurs when patients are taking high doses of steroids for long periods of time. Avascular necrosis occurs when there is loss of normal blood flow to the center of the bone. This usually occurs in the hips (femoral head) or the shoulders (humeral head). Patients report a great deal of pain and an MRI shows that avascular necrosis has occurred.

Potential side effects of steroids

Increased risk of infections at high doses of steroids
Higher blood sugar and diabetes
Stomach ulcers, especially when used with NSAIDs
Osteoporosis
High blood pressure
Worsening of congestive heart failure
Insomnia and mood changes
Weight gain and increased appetite
Adrenal insufficiency
Easy bruising, skin fragility, delayed wound healing

> Muscle weakness and atrophy
>
> Cushing syndrome and moon facies
>
> Cataracts and glaucoma
>
> Avascular necrosis
>
> Acne

Can steroid injections into my joints be harmful for them over time?

Some patients receive steroid injections into the knees, shoulders, or other joints to help with symptoms and reduce flares. Certain research studies have shown that using too many steroid injections over several years can cause accelerated degeneration of the cartilage within joints. It's unclear whether this was a direct result of the steroid itself, or whether patients felt better after the injection and became more active with increased wear-and-tear on the joints and cartilage.

Due to the findings from research studies, it is not recommended to perform steroid injections into any joint more often than once every 3-4 months. Some guidelines recommend no more than 2-3 steroid injections into a joint per year.

Are steroids safe to take during pregnancy and breastfeeding?

Research studies have shown that taking prednisone and other steroids during pregnancy can increase fetal harm and cause low birth weight or birth defects. There is an increased incidence of cleft lip or cleft palate when steroids are taken during the first trimester of pregnancy.

Steroids are usually avoided during pregnancy unless a mom is really suffering and doesn't have other options for pain control. Steroids can also reduce breast milk supply and is usually avoided during the postpartum period.

Can I receive vaccines while taking a steroid?

Yes, you can receive any vaccine that is an <u>inactivated</u> vaccine—such as the flu shot, new shingles shot, and other inactive ones. Avoid <u>live vaccines</u> such as the flu nasal mist and the measles/mumps/rubella vaccine.

Will steroids blunt my immune system's response to vaccines?

There is evidence that the immune system doesn't respond as well to vaccinations while under the influence of steroids. If you want to maximize and optimize your immune system's response to a vaccine—for example the COVID-19 vaccine—you could try stopping your steroid and other immunosuppressants before receiving the vaccine.

This will be discussed more in chapter 9, "Navigating rheumatoid arthritis during the COVID-19 pandemic."

Summary of steroid medications:

Prednisone and other steroids are usually used temporarily for arthritis flares or when a patient is first diagnosed and is waiting for long-term medications to build up to therapeutic levels. They have a lot of side effects and shouldn't be taken long-term. The less steroid, the better!

Case scenarios

These case scenarios are illustrations of journeys that different patients may experience, which are loosely based on the paths that some of my patients have taken with steroid medications. Names have been changed for anonymity.

Case 1

Ed has occasional flares of his rheumatoid arthritis and takes a prednisone taper when he has increased symptoms caused by weather changes or increased levels of stress. He has a supply of prednisone tablets at home to keep on hand for occasional flares. He only takes 1-2 prednisone courses per year lasting about 2 weeks each time, and otherwise feels good on his regular rheumatoid arthritis medication regimen.

Case 2

Theresa takes prednisone 5 mg daily as a regular part of her rheumatoid arthritis regimen. She has done this for several years ever since her initial diagnosis of rheumatoid arthritis. When her previous rheumatologist retired and she established care with a new rheumatologist, she was told that weaning down on her dose of prednisone and stopping it eventually would be the best course of action, since she has osteoporosis and prednisone weakens her bones even more.

Theresa was really surprised to hear this from her new rheumatologist, and a bit taken aback. She was hoping to continue the same medications and just get some refills from her new doctor. After doing some reading about osteoporosis and steroid side effects, she agreed to cut down on prednisone. She was able to wean down on prednisone slowly by 1 mg each month until finally reaching zero and stopping completely.

Case 3

Benjamin is 95 years old and has lived a long time with rheumatoid arthritis, ever since the 1980s when he used to receive gold injections for his arthritis. He takes prednisone 2 mg daily and can tell the difference if he doesn't take it, even though it's a low dose. At 95 years old, he and his rheumatologist decided that it's more about quality of life at this point and less about the long-term side effects of medications.

Ben wants to live with less pain in the present moment and isn't as worried about side effects in the future such as osteoporosis, diabetes, and weight gain. He and his rheumatologist decide together that he will continue the prednisone because benefits outweigh the risks.

OVER-THE-COUNTER MEDICATIONS

What are common medications I can find over-the-counter to help with my arthritis pain?

Common over-the-counter medications are Tylenol, Advil, or Aleve. Patients are typically taking some of these medications when they first come to see me as a rheumatologist, and as they start to feel better with the long-term treatments, they are able to wean down on how much over-the-counter medications they are taking.

What is the main difference between Tylenol (acetaminophen) and Advil (ibuprofen)? Do they have different side effects?

Whereas Tylenol mostly works by inhibiting pain receptors in the central nervous system or brain, Advil works more to reduce inflammatory mediators within the joints and other peripheral tissues themselves. Tylenol relieves pain and fevers, but is not known to reduce inflammation to any significant degree. Advil relieves pain, fever, and has an effect on inflammation in tissues to a certain extent. A lot of patients tend to say that Advil works much better than Tylenol for their joint pain and stiffness.

Tylenol is known to have a better safety profile and fewer side effects than Advil. If you stay within the recommended dosage of less than 4000 mg of Tylenol per day, it should be safe for your liver, unless you have underlying liver disease. Tylenol does not usually cause stomach upset or kidney problems.

Mechanism of Action

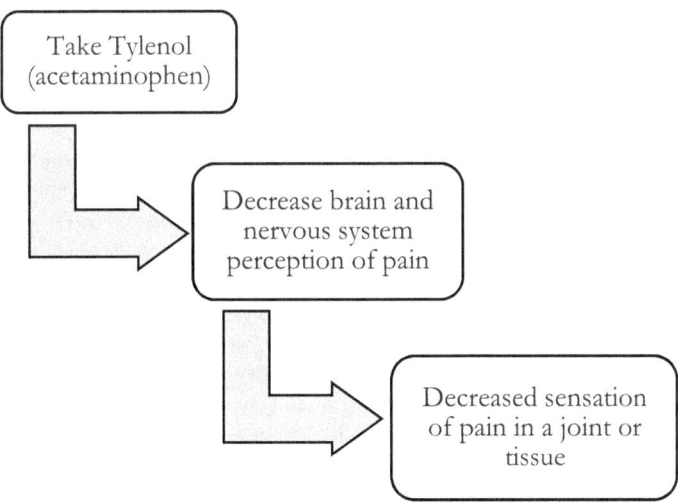

On the other hand, NSAID medications like Advil can cause stomach upset, ulcers, or renal insufficiency. We usually see this in patients who take high doses of Advil over long periods of time. Taking a little Advil once in a while shouldn't be a major issue, but definitely avoid it if you have underlying health problems like stomach ulcers, high blood pressure, coronary artery disease, congestive heart failure, or kidney failure.

Advil can make heart disease such as coronary artery disease or congestive heart failure worse. Advil can also have drug interactions with blood thinners and make you bruise or bleed more easily, because it affects how the platelets (cells in the bloodstream and that cause clotting and stop bleeding) work in your body.

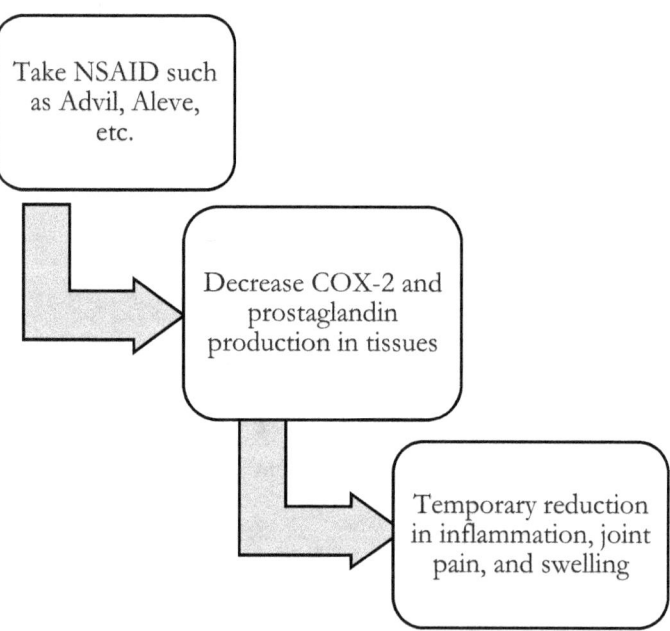

Potential side effects of Tylenol versus Advil/Aleve

Tylenol	Advil/Aleve/NSAIDs
Liver damage if too high doses	Stomach upset or pain
Worsening of underlying liver diseases	Stomach ulcers
Interference with certain blood glucose monitors (reported by patients)	Worsening of congestive heart failure
	Salt retention
	Kidney damage
	Increased risk of heart attack or stroke
	Increased bruising or bleeding
	Drug interactions with blood thinners

What are NSAID medications that are similar to Advil, or ibuprofen?

The NSAID family of medications, which stands for "non-steroid anti-inflammatory drugs," include a large number of medications that are similar to Advil or Aleve. They all work through similar receptors in the body to have the same ultimate effects of reducing pain and inflammation. A few of them are found over-the-counter and the rest are prescriptions.

Please note that **Celebrex (celecoxib)** is different from the other NSAIDs in that it tends to have fewer side effects on the stomach. We typically use Celebrex in patients with a history of stomach ulcers or stomach upset from previous use of other NSAIDS. It can still cause side effects on the digestive tract, but there is less risk compared to the other NSAIDs.

Brand name	Generic name	Prescription or Over-the-counter (OTC)
Advil	Ibuprofen	OTC
Aleve	Naproxen	OTC
Motrin	Ibuprofen	OTC
Naprosyn	Naproxen	OTC
Mobic	Meloxicam	Prescription
Feldene	Piroxicam	Prescription
Indocin	Indomethacin	Prescription
Celebrex	Celecoxib	Prescription
Voltaren	Diclofenac	Prescription
Lodine	Etodolac	Prescription
Relafen	Nabumetone	Prescription
Toradol	Ketorolac	Prescription
Clinoril	Sulindac	Prescription

Are there any topical creams or ointments I can rub on my joints for pain relief?

A great topical medication that was previously prescription-only and just became available over-the-counter is Voltaren gel, also known as diclofenac 1% topical gel. This is a topical NSAID that you can rub directly on your painful joints rather than taking a pill.

The benefit of using this topical gel is that it has very little absorption into your system, less than 7%, which means less side effects for your body. The package insert says to be careful using it if you have heart or kidney conditions, but due to the low systemic absorption, the likelihood that it would cause organ damage is extremely low.

I have seen mixed results with the topical Voltaren gel. Some patients say it works really well and they love it, but others say it hardly does anything at all. Some patients say it can be inconvenient to put on areas like the hand joints, because they have to use their hands or wash them, which isn't very practical. In any case, Voltaren topical gel isn't very expensive or harmful, so it is worth a try.

Here are some other topical ointments to try:

- Biofreeze and icy hot: camphor and menthol
- Aspercreme: Capsaicin
- Lidocaine
- Australian dream
- Tiger balm
- Blue emu and Salon Pas

Will over-the-counter medications help prevent joint damage over time, or are they more of a temporary band-aid over the underlying issue?

Over-the-counter medications are just a temporary band-aid for joint pain. Even though the name "NSAID" implies that some degree of inflammation is being blocked, medications like Advil and Aleve won't address the underlying autoimmune process going on in your body.

Tylenol and Advil are not strong enough to prevent joint damage and deformities from occurring over the years. They have also caused serious side effects, especially Advil, Aleve, and other NSAIDs causing gastrointestinal bleeding and kidney damage. Even though DMARDs, biologics, and Jak inhibitors also have potential side effects, they address the underlying autoimmune process and have long-term efficacy in protecting the joints.

What can I take for sleep that is over-the-counter?

For myself, I take melatonin 5 mg or 10 mg once in a while if I have trouble falling asleep. Melatonin has the least side effects and is a natural hormone-derived sleep aid.

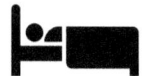

I haven't found that I feel groggier the next day or that my mood is any different with taking melatonin (although note that there is always a disclaimer on the bottle for patients with depression). I have also seen some brands that contain melatonin with L-theanine and valerian root, which are homeopathic and herbal sleep aids.

Younger patients can occasionally take Advil PM or Tylenol PM for pain and sleep. The "PM" part usually means it contains diphenhydramine, which is the same thing as generic Benadryl. Benadryl is for allergies, but also makes people feel sedated and sleepy.

Older patients above age 65 should avoid medications like Benadryl, Tylenol PM, or Advil PM. In elderly patients, diphenhydramine can cause confusion, dry mouth, bladder retention, or other side effects.

Sleep hygiene is also important for reducing mind-body noise in preparation for sleep. It is a list of basic behavioral and environmental changes that can help you sleep better:

- Establish the bedroom as a stress-free and work-free sanctuary.

- Limit exposure to stressful imagery from your phone, television, and radio.
- Don't watch the clock.
- Sleep in total darkness or use a sleep mask.
- Maintain a regular sleep-wake cycle.
- Avoid napping during the daytime.
- Avoid caffeine and exercise prior to bedtime.

Further discussion on fatigue and sleep will be in the next section on holistic, natural, and complementary management strategies for rheumatoid arthritis.

Case scenarios

These case scenarios are illustrations of journeys that different patients may experience, which are loosely based on the paths that some of my patients have taken with NSAIDs and over-the-counter medications. Names have been changed for anonymity.

Case 1

David usually takes Advil twice a day for his arthritis pain, along with methotrexate and Humira as part of his treatment regimen. He recently had his 3-month lab work checked and it showed that his kidneys aren't working as well as they did when he was younger. His rheumatologist and his primary care doctor both advise him to cut down on his Advil intake for the sake of his kidneys.

His rheumatologist adjusts his dose of methotrexate slightly so that he doesn't have to take Advil as often. At the next blood draw, his labs show that his kidney function is stable or slightly improving.

Case 2

Kristen tried taking ibuprofen and Aleve for arthritis pain, but had stomach upset and terrible acid reflux with both. Her rheumatologist prescribed Celebrex instead, and Kristen found it to be easier on the stomach and digestive tract.

Case 3

Laura used to take Advil for flares of joint pain or occasional migraines. Recently she was diagnosed with atrial fibrillation and was started on blood thinners. She is no longer able to take Advil because of drug interactions with the blood thinners, and Tylenol doesn't work for her at all.

Laura tried the topical Voltaren gel and rubs it on her knees and wrists at night before bedtime to help with pain. She also receives a referral to a pain management specialist because is stuck with not having a lot of good options for pain control.

Action list:

- ☐ Make a list of what over-the-counter medications you are taking, and at what doses.

- ☐ Make a note of any side effects you are experiencing from these medications, such as stomach upset.

- ☐ Make a note of any reasons to avoid over-the-counter Tylenol, Advil, or the other ones listed in this chapter. For example, a history of stomach ulcers or kidney failure could be reasons to avoid Advil.

- ☐ Make a list of any other questions you have for your rheumatologist about any over-the-counter medications you are taking.

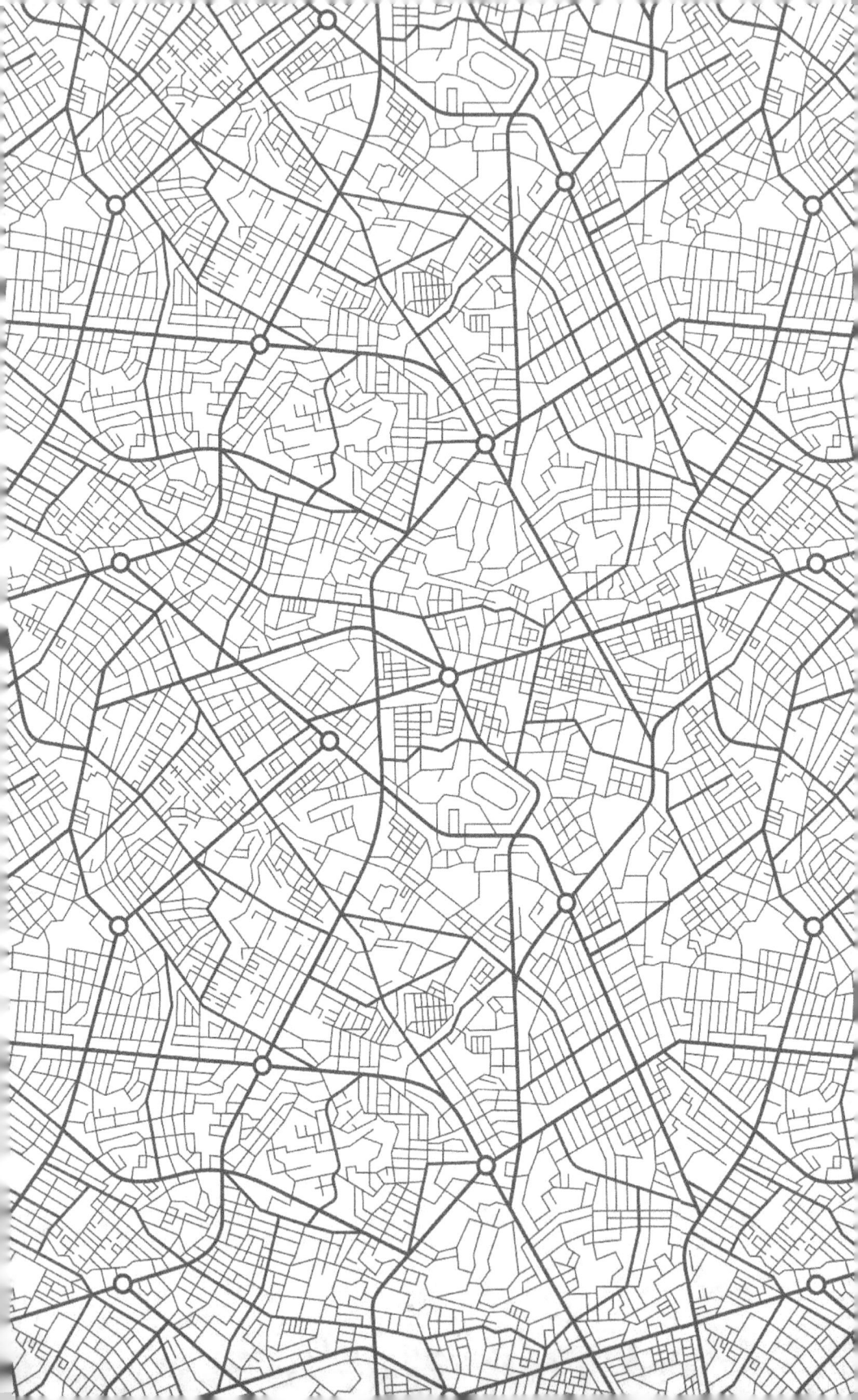

CHAPTER 7

NAVIGATING HOLISTIC, NATURAL, AND COMPLEMENTARY APPROACHES TO RHEUMATOID ARTHRITIS

AN INTEGRATIVE APPROACH TO RHEUMATOID ARTHRITIS

"When one tugs at a single thing in nature, he finds it attached to the rest of the world." [John Muir]

An integrative approach is taking the entire body and "whole health" into account, rather than treating each body part as a separate disconnected entity. Integrative medicine honors the intricate connection between, mind, body, and spirit, and stays open-minded towards natural and holistic approaches to managing chronic pain and fatigue.

Instead of just focusing on prescription medications and invasive procedures like joint surgery, this approach takes multiple viewpoints in the spectrum of heath maintenance into consideration, and works collaboratively with other disciplines such as chiropractics, Eastern medicine, or complementary treatments. Lifestyle interventions such as nutrition, dietary changes, exercise, and stress reduction are also important pieces of integrative medicine.

The benefit of integrative medicine is that it can more closely match a patient's individual beliefs, culture, and preferences about his or her own health. It can also help with minimizing expensive healthcare costs and delay the need for more invasive measures such as surgery. The challenge or drawback of this approach is making sure that holistic therapies are evidence-based and safe for patients. Looking at research studies and strength of recommendations can help prevent both patients and doctors from buying into fraudulent claims.

While prescription medications are extensively researched and stringently regulated by the FDA, there are no quality or safety measures in place to monitor alternative therapies, which can result in unclear benefits and side effects of these treatments. This means that doctors and patients usually have to do more of their own research in understanding these treatments.

An integrative approach also emphasizes shared decision-making with patients, active listening on the part of the physician, and open-mindedness to the patient's preferences, cultural beliefs, and perspectives regarding their health. The patient should be an active partner who plays a vital role in health and healing.

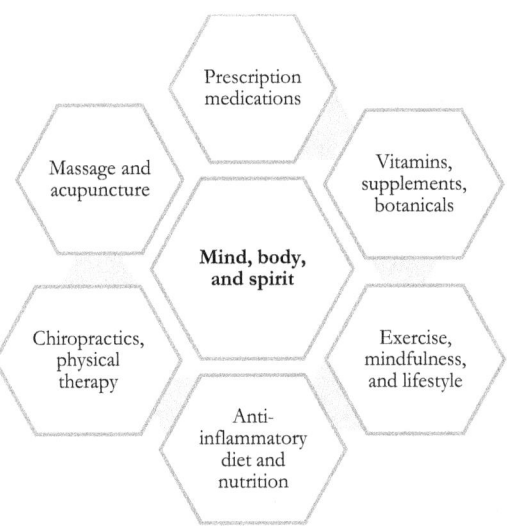

Can my rheumatoid arthritis be managed through holistic and alternative strategies alone?

It's possible, and I have a few patients who are using natural methods instead of taking prescription medications. They keep a very strict anti-inflammatory diet and treat occasional flares of their arthritis with a prednisone taper.

Overall, most of my patients are taking a multifaceted and integrative approach to their rheumatoid arthritis management. They are taking one or two prescription medications, as well as trying their best with eating healthy, and reducing flares as much possible. Being proactive with medications may be needed for patients with aggressive or severe rheumatoid arthritis that requires more heavy-duty treatments, as opposed to milder arthritis that can be managed by natural methods alone.

In the end, it's *your* body and you should do whatever you feel is the best fit for yourself, whether that be taking medications and/or trying more of a natural approach. Myself, I sit at the intersection between Eastern and Western medicine. I have seen extremes from both ends of the spectrum—my mom believes wholeheartedly in Chinese medicine and abides by natural treatments and supplements only. She doesn't even like to go see doctors.

During my career, I have also met doctors who don't believe in natural methods at all because they don't feel that there's enough research behind certain claims. They are on the opposite side of the spectrum in believing only in Western medicine and prescriptions approved by the FDA.

Having seen both sides of the coin, I tend to support my patients no matter which route they'd like to take. The only caveat is when a patient already has joint damage that has occurred from aggressive rheumatoid arthritis. In that circumstance, I advise a more proactive strategy and try to start a prescription medication early on to prevent further joint damage from occurring.

What are natural vitamins, botanicals, and supplements I can take to help me with my rheumatoid arthritis?

- Turmeric: an anti-inflammatory spice that we discussed in chapter 2. Turmeric contains curcumin which is the active component to reduce inflammation by blocking COX-2, an inflammatory substance in the body.
- Ginger: also an anti-inflammatory spice.
- Glucosamine and chondroitin supplements: mostly studied in osteoarthritis with mixed results. Some studies show effectiveness in osteoarthritis and other studies show no significant difference.
- Fish oil and omega-3 fatty acids.
- Borage oil: contains gamma-linolenic acid which is an omega-6 fatty acid that can reduce inflammation.
- Boswellia serrata: also known as Indian frankincense, there is a gum resin derived from this plant that has anti-inflammatory properties in the body.
- Cat's claw: plant from South American rainforests with anti-inflammatory properties that help with joint pain, swelling, and morning joint stiffness.
- Probiotics to help with gut and digestive health.
- Green tea: high in catechins that reduce inflammatory activity.

How do I use heat and cold therapy?

Heat is known to increase blood flow to an area, whereas cold therapy is known to decrease inflammation and swelling around tissues. Patients often use both heat and cold, sometimes alternating them, to help with pain relief.

Hot baths and showers can relieve morning joint stiffness. Paraffin wax baths for the hands and feet can feel extremely soothing for joint pain. Applying heat is also known to raise the body's pain threshold and help with muscle relaxation.

Cold therapy can be used when a joint is swollen or red to reduce inflammation. Ice packs are sometimes used after exercise to relieve muscle aching and pain after working out. Avoid using heat or cold therapy on areas where you have abnormal sensation—for example, peripheral neuropathy of the feet.

What are Synvisc injections?

Synvisc is an injectable form of hyaluronic acid, one of the components of cartilage. Synvisc has been studied in the management of knee osteoarthritis. The idea of the injections is to support cartilage health and increase lubrication within the joints to improve mobility and decrease pain. Results from studies were mixed, with some patients reporting a significant improvement and other patients experiencing no difference compared to placebo.

What is the role of stem cell therapy in rheumatoid arthritis?

The idea behind stem cell therapy is that stem cells can become any type of cell in the body. Some believe that stem cells can help regenerate cartilage and other tissues within joints that have been worn out with use over time. This sounds like a brilliant concept, but research studies have not fully substantiated the claims of stem cell therapy.

Since it has not been proven to be significantly better than placebo, stem cell therapy is not covered by insurance and tends to be quite expensive. Some patients have paid on their own to receive this therapy and said it really helped, so I believe the results are on a case-by-case basis with mixed reports.

What is the role of platelet rich plasma in rheumatoid arthritis?

Platelet rich plasma (PRP) is derived from the patient's own blood, which has been spun down. The plasma component is taken out and separated from the red blood cells. The plasma contains components in the blood that are involved with tissue healing.

Similar to stem cell therapy, research hasn't fully substantiated the effects of platelet rich plasma. It tends to be an expensive treatment that is not covered by insurance. Results are mixed with some patients saying it was helpful and others saying it didn't do anything for their pain.

What is the role of chiropractors in rheumatoid arthritis?

Chiropractors can adjust and evaluate the spine and other joints for proper alignment. They can perform adjustments on the spine to realign it back to a proper position. Chiropractic manipulations can help with chronic neck pain, back pain, and other symptoms.

What is the role of massage therapy in rheumatoid arthritis?

Massage therapists can help with myofascial pain, which is pain in the muscles and soft tissues. They can feel areas of tension in the muscles and ligaments. One study showed that Swedish massage helped patients who were experiencing pain from osteoarthritis. Massage therapy can also help with relaxation, stress reduction, meditation, mindfulness, and other important aspects of self-care. It also promotes healthy blood flow and release of neurotransmitters that fight depression and anxiety.

What is the role of acupuncture or acupressure in rheumatoid arthritis?

Acupuncture and acupressure both have roots in Eastern medicine, originating from ancient China. By stimulating certain areas of the superficial body that correlate with deeper organs and components of the nervous system, these practices are thought to encourage the body's own healing process.

In research trials done on the effects of acupuncture, there were increased levels of endorphins and neurotransmitters detected in patients undergoing acupuncture. Studies also showed improvement in pain levels and fatigue compared to placebo or "sham" treatments. For example, acupuncture was approved by the United Kingdom's National Institute for Health and Care Excellence for treating chronic low back pain because research studies showed that it is less expensive, less invasive, and had longer-lasting effects compared to epidural steroid injections for treatment of chronic low back pain.

What is the role of Ayurvedic medicine in rheumatoid arthritis?

Ayurvedic medicine has deep roots in India. In Ayurvedic teaching, there are five elements—air, fire, water, earth, and space—that can determine a patient's bodily humour or constitutional state of being. For example, a state of excess "pitta" indicates increased fire or inflammation within the body. Certain foods, herbs, exercises, and lifestyle changes may pacify imbalanced pitta states.

For example, ashwagandha is an Ayurvedic herb that is also known as Indian ginseng. Ashwagandha has anti-inflammatory, antioxidant, anxiolytic, and antidepressant activity in the body. It is used to lower stress and regulate the nervous system. Regular meditation, sufficient sleep, retreats, and relaxation also help with pitta states.

What is the role of reiki energy healing in rheumatoid arthritis?

Reiki energy healing has roots in Japan, and is based on the idea that all living beings have an invisible magnetic field surrounding their bodies and subtle energy force emanating from their beings. Although it can sound mystical or unbelievable, there have been studies done on sharks showing that they can sense the magnetic fields of their prey and other living beings in the ocean. Even if the sharks can't visibly see other fish and living creatures in the water, they are aware of their presence because of these magnetic fields.

Reiki practices describe how a person's magnetic and energy field can become disturbed or out of alignment, leading to various ailments and symptoms. The role of reiki energy healers is to help a person's energy force and magnetic field come back to a healthy alignment, thus helping with the body's own natural healing process.

What we can learn from other cultures about whole health and healing:

Indian culture	• Ayurvedic medicine • Yoga • Turmeric
Chinese culture	• Acupuncture • Tai chi • Traditional Chinese medicine
Japanese culture	• Reiki energy healing • Okinawan diet • Meditation, mindfulness
South American cultures	• Botanicals and herbs

What is the role of aromatherapy in rheumatoid arthritis?

Aromatherapy is using natural ointments from essential oils to help with stress, headaches, insomnia, anxiety, fatigue, and other symptoms. Lavender is one of the most widely used scents to promote peace, calm, and relaxation.

Peppermint oil has been used for headaches, fatigue, and sinus problems. Patients have mentioned that essential oils have helped them with sleep issues and depression, which can often coexist with rheumatoid arthritis.

Is CBD cream or oil used for rheumatoid arthritis?

CBD oil doesn't contain THC, which is the substance that gets people "high" when they smoke, vape, or eat marijuana. Since CBD oil doesn't influence the brain that way, some patients have tried it for pain and sleep. CBD oil affects two receptors, called cannabinoid receptor 1 and 2, and is still being studied in chronic pain conditions such as rheumatoid arthritis.

A few studies done with CBD oil in patients with rheumatoid arthritis did show that they had reduced levels of pain and could sleep better. CBD oil usually comes as a capsule or in liquid drops. Possible side effects include nausea, fatigue, diarrhea, headaches, or appetite changes. The purity of CBD oil from certain vendors is not regulated or monitored.

Is medical marijuana used for rheumatoid arthritis?

With medical marijuana now being legal in more than half the states in America, a lot of patients are asking about whether they can use marijuana to treat the chronic pain with their rheumatoid arthritis. Marijuana can affect the neurotransmitters involved in the cycle of chronic pain.

However, the anti-inflammatory activity of cannabis is still being studied. Whereas medications like DMARDs, biologics, and the JAK inhibitors alter the course and progression of the disease, it's unknown whether marijuana would stop joint damage from occurring.

I have a few patients using medical marijuana when they don't have other good options for pain control. For example, Tylenol doesn't work on everyone, some can't take ibuprofen or other NSAIDs because of side effects, and some want to avoid opioid narcotics. Some doctors (but not all) have a license to prescribe medical marijuana on a case-by-case basis.

What is a TENS unit?

A transcutaneous electrical nerve stimulation (TENS) unit has been studied in various painful conditions, including arthritis, fibromyalgia, and peripheral neuropathy. The concept behind how it works is actually very similar to how acupuncture is hypothesized to work. By stimulating superficial nerves, the nervous system releases endorphins and neurotransmitters to help with pain.

What are natural products I can use for insomnia and better sleep?

- Melatonin
- L-theanine
- Valerian root
- Lavender essential oil
- CBD oil
- Lemon balm
- Calming herbs such as chamomile
- Mindfulness, meditation, progressive muscle relaxation, focused breathing exercises, and guided imagery

What is sleep hygiene?

Sleep hygiene is important for reducing mind-body noise in preparation for sleep. It is a list of basic behavioral and environmental changes that can help you sleep better:

- Establish the bedroom as a stress-free and work-free sanctuary.

- Limit exposure to stressful imagery from your phone, television, and radio. Avoid exposure to blue lights from screens prior to sleep.
- Don't watch the clock. Conceal clocks if possible.
- Sleep in total darkness or use a sleep mask.
- Maintain a regular sleep-wake cycle, even on the weekends.
- Avoid napping during the daytime.
- Avoid caffeine and exercise prior to bedtime.
- Make sure the temperature in the bedroom is right for you—not too hot or too cold.

What are some natural topical ointments or rubs I can use for rheumatoid arthritis?

- Biofreeze and icy hot: contain camphor and menthol
- Aspercreme: contains capsaicin
- Lidocaine
- Australian dream
- Tiger balm
- Blue emu
- Salon pas

What is the connection between mind, body, and spirit in maintaining health and wellness?

Aristotle believed that every person was a combination of both physical and spiritual properties with no separation between mind and body. I wholeheartedly agree that all parts of the body are intricately connected. Everything that affects your physical body will affect your mind and spirit, and vice versa. By taking care of your mental and spiritual health, you are providing a better environment for your body to undergo healing and achieve optimal vitality.

One manifestation of the mind and body connection that I see quite often in my patients is the *chronic cognitive-emotional hyperarousal syndrome*, which I mentioned in a previous chapter. As a result of previous  trauma, chronic pain, or chronic stress, the body can enter a "fight or flight" mode with chronic activation of the sympathetic nervous system that is difficult to shut off. The primitive amygdala in the brain retains stressful memories that stimulate the nervous system when the body and mind perceive stress, danger, and pain.

As a result of the imbalance between the sympathetic ("fight or flight") and parasympathetic ("rest and digest") nervous systems, patients can experience a multitude of symptoms affecting almost every body part. When your body enters "survival mode," you can feel your muscles tensing up involuntarily, heart pounding, rapid and shallow breathing, and stomach clenching up. Over time, this can cause chronic headaches or migraines, chest pain and trouble breathing, irritable bowel and bladder symptoms, fatigue, anxiety, and insomnia, to name a few.

As one patient put it, she is "hypervigilant and extremely sensitive to any symptoms in her body" and "has a lot of anxiety about symptoms that could mean something is wrong with her body." There is an excellent book on this topic called "The Body Keeps the Score: Brain, Mind, and Body in the Healing of Trauma," by Dr. Bessel Van Der Kolk, which I highly recommend to anyone who wants to understand more about the process of chronic pain.

To escape the chronic cognitive-emotional hyperarousal syndrome, we have to teach our bodies to turn off its fight or flight mode in a gentle way. We have to show ourselves that despite the stresses and anxiety of modern life, we are not being chased by a saber-toothed tiger. The "tiger" could be a ruthless boss or a financial burden, but the danger we perceive is not necessarily life-threatening in most cases.

Slowly, we find healthy ways of processing the anxiety and worries of everyday life so that they don't worsen our well-being or manifest in physical symptoms such as chronic fatigue or a vicious chronic pain cycle.

What are some exercises I can participate in to promote a healthier connection between my mind, body, and spirit?

- Meditation and mindfulness: practice being present with *what is* in silence and stillness, rather than letting your mind drift to the past, future, or other concerns. Maintain a fluid awareness of moment-by-moment experiences in a nonjudgmental and nonreactive way.

  Let everything be as it is without trying to change anything. Accept the present moment for what it is, not as something good or bad. If your mind drifts, simply guide it back to the present moment without criticizing yourself.

- Journaling: has been shown to help patients cope with pain related to rheumatoid arthritis. In one study, patients with rheumatoid arthritis who wrote about stressful events showed a 28% reduction in disease severity compared to those who did not participate in journaling. Similar improvements were seen in patients with asthma who journaled.

  Expressive writing was also shown to improve memory capacity, cognitive functioning, and decrease rates of depression and anxiety. These are excellent results considering that no medications were needed, only a pen, paper, and a chunk of time. Write down stressful events, as well as things you are grateful for.

- Yoga nidra: a branch of yoga that teaches stillness, rest, letting go, and mind-body relaxation. I highly recommend the book "Radiant Rest: Yoga Nidra for Deep Relaxation and Awakened Clarity" by Tracee Stanley.

- Tai chi: combines elements of martial arts and meditative movements that promote balance and healing of the mind and body. Postures are performed slowly and flow into one another. Tai chi has been shown to improve balance, muscle relaxation, breathing, concentration, and mental health.

- Deep breathing and biofeedback
- Music therapy

How can we tell which alternative therapies have enough evidence or research to back up their claims?

You can use the "strength of recommendation taxonomy" (SORT) rating which grades the therapies on a scale:

- Grade A: consistent, good-quality, patient-oriented evidence. For example, acupuncture has an A grading for being an alternative treatment for nausea and vomiting because there is quality research supporting this.

- Grade B: inconsistent or limited-quality evidence. For example, taking ginger has a B grading for treating pain associated with osteoarthritis.
- Grade C: only expert opinion, consensus, and usual practice guidelines are available. No formal research studies available.

How can we tell which alternative therapies could be potentially harmful?

You can use the grading scale for harm to determine whether therapies pose any risk:

- Grade 3: most harm and potential to result in death or permanent disability. For example, the botanical supplement *Aristolochia* (birthwort) has the potential to cause cancer.
- Grade 2: moderate harm with the potential to cause reversible side effects or drug interactions.
- Grade 1: least harm with little, if any, risk of dangerous effects. For example, eating an anti-inflammatory diet.

Case scenarios

These case scenarios are illustrations of journeys that different patients may experience, which are loosely based on the paths that some of my patients have taken with holistic, natural, and alternative approaches for rheumatoid arthritis. Names have been changed for anonymity.

Case 1

Sherry sees her rheumatologist on a regular basis for office visits, and takes her rheumatoid arthritis medications as prescribed. She also sees a holistic and complementary doctor at a natural health clinic. She has a list of about 15 supplements that the holistic doctor recommended for her. Sherry also uses CBD oil at night before bed to help her sleep. She feels that these vitamins and supplements are a helpful adjunctive therapy for her rheumatoid arthritis.

Case 2

Sara has her rheumatoid arthritis under good control, but she experiences a lot of chronic lower back pain from degenerative disc disease. She doesn't feel ready to see a pain management doctor for steroid injections into the lower back and sought advice from a chiropractor instead. Her chiropractor told her that her spine and hips are out of alignment and he adjusted them to a better position.

There is also an acupuncturist at the chiropractor's office who performed acupuncture on Sara to help with her chronic low back pain. Overall, she feels that the adjustments and acupuncture treatments are very helpful for her lower back pain while being minimally invasive, and she continues to receive them every 3 months or so.

Case 3

Adam feels that his joint pain and swelling have resolved after starting his rheumatoid arthritis treatment, but the main symptoms he's dealing with now is severe fatigue and exhaustion. He feels really tired all day at work and is ready to take a nap after work. He doesn't have like he has enough energy to devote to his wife and children.

Adam decided to see an alternative doctor for additional advice for his fatigue. He got hair strand testing done which showed that he was low in magnesium, and the naturopathic doctor recommended that he take some magnesium supplements. He also had food testing done and found out that his body doesn't tolerate or react well to a number of commonplace foods and ingredients, such as bananas and tomatoes. He cut these foods out of his diet and is going to see if his energy levels improve.

Action list:

- ☐ Make a list of vitamins and supplements you are interested in trying.

- ☐ Do more research and reading into complementary and alternative strategies that may be a good fit for you.

- ☐ Start doing one activity that will promote a healthy connection with your mind, body, and spirit.

- ☐ Prioritize self-care and schedule a massage or other relaxing activity this week.

- ☐ Brainstorm ways to reduce stress and anxiety in your life.

Reflection questions:

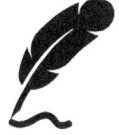

1. Which of the complementary practices seem to be a good fit for you?

2. Which of the alternative strategies would you like to do more reading and research about?

3. Do you have any opinion on medical marijuana and CBD products, either positive or negative?

4. Do you pay much attention to the mind-body-spirit connection? Why or why not?

5. Have you ever felt the effects of the chronic cognitive-emotional hyperarousal syndrome? If so, how has it affected you?

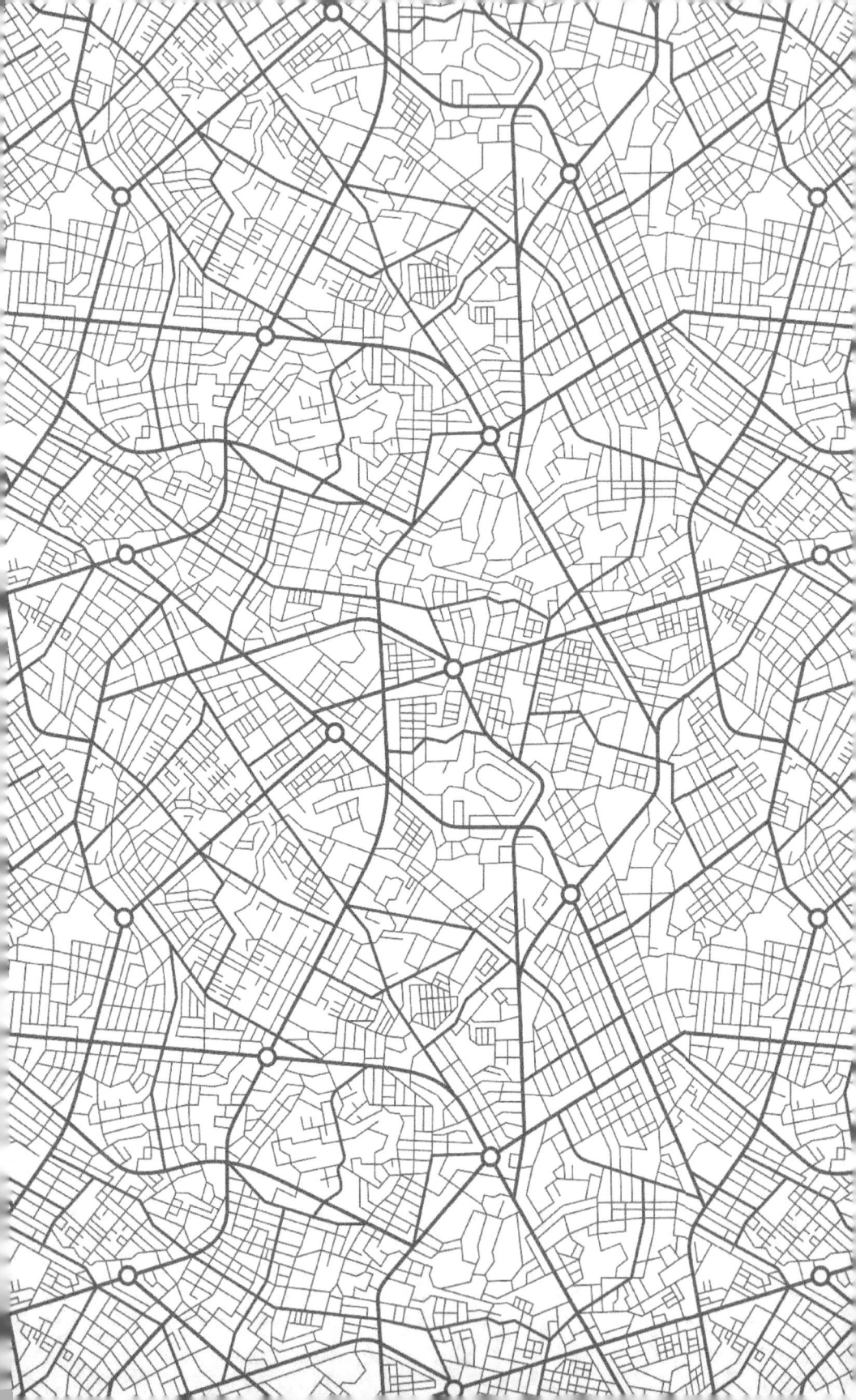

CHAPTER 8

NAVIGATING EXERCISE, PHYSICAL THERAPY, SURGERY, AND ASSISTIVE AIDS

EXERCISING WITH RHEUMATOID ARTHRITIS

What are benefits of exercise in rheumatoid arthritis?

- Reduce joint stiffness. "A body in motion stays in motion."
- Maintain muscle mass and prevent muscle atrophy. "If you don't use it, you lose it."
- Maintain bone mass and reduce risk of osteoporosis and bone fractures. Patients with rheumatoid arthritis have a higher risk of developing osteoporosis. You can help maintain your bone mass by staying active and getting enough calcium and vitamin D in your diet.
- Reduce biomechanical load that the joints are carrying every day by maintaining a healthy weight. The joints are very sensitive to weight. For every 4 kg of weight gain, the biomechanical load on the joints increases by about four-fold, leading to increased wear and tear on your joints.
- Maintain balance and agility.
- Reduce inflammation in the body.
- Reduce stress and anxiety.
- Improve sleep and fatigue.
- Improve cardiovascular health.
- Maintain brain and neurological health. Patients who exercise have been found to maintain their brain volume, and exercise has preventative effects against Alzheimer's dementia and memory deterioration.

What are recommended forms of exercise for patients with rheumatoid arthritis?

Low weight-bearing exercises are recommended because they exert less wear and tear on the joints.

- Elliptical
- Recumbent or stationary bicycling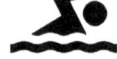
- Rowing machine
- Swimming and water aerobics
- Walking
- Light weight lifting
- Yoga
- Tai chi

Can yoga be beneficial for patients with rheumatoid arthritis?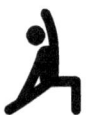

Yes, yoga can be anything from light stretching and meditation to a heavy muscle-toning and aerobic workout. Yoga can be tailored to each individual's needs and lifestyle. It can be suitable for those who can't do heavy workouts like running or jogging. It can help maintain muscle mass and stretch tendons and ligaments.

Yoga also reduces stress and promotes a healthy mind-body-spirit connection. A helpful book called "Yoga for Arthritis: The Complete Guide" by Loren Fishman and Ellen Saltonstall can teach you to do yoga in a safe way for your joints.

Can tai chi be beneficial for patients with rheumatoid arthritis?

Tai chi combines elements of martial arts and meditative movements that promote balance and healing of the mind and body. Postures are performed slowly and flow into one another. Tai chi has been shown to improve balance, muscle relaxation, breathing, concentration, and mental health.

How do I get the right balance between exercising enough but not pushing my body too far to cause a flare?

- Listen to your body.
- Establish a gradual exercise program.
- Alternate activities on different days.
- Schedule days of rest.

What if I absolutely cannot exercise due to severe pain and fatigue? What if exercise actually makes me feel worse?

Some people have really tried hard at exercise and it's just not their thing. They may even feel much worse after they exercise. Some patients have told me that if they feel good one day and try to exercise or get a lot of chores done around the house, they're "down for the next week with severe pain and fatigue and can't even get out of bed."

If you feel unable to exercise, at least do some stretching once or twice a day. Do something that does make your body feel good, like giving your muscles and joints a massage. There is a book called "Stretching to Stay Young" by Jessica Matthews, which I highly recommend to anyone who can't do more strenuous exercises.

PHYSICAL THERAPY

What is the role of physical therapy in rheumatoid arthritis?

- Build strength of the structures around joints such as muscles, tendons, ligaments.
- Reduce pain and increase mobility and functionality of joints.
- Improve range of motion of joints.
- Reduce scar tissue development after joint injuries.
- Learn safe ways of using joints, for example, how to lift a heavy box without injuring your lower back.
- Learn home exercises to do on your own after therapy sessions end.
- Identify any need for assistive devices such as canes or walkers.
- Help with recovery and ambulation after surgeries.

What is the role of occupational therapy in rheumatoid arthritis?

- Learn how to approach activities of daily living, such as bathing, getting dressed, and cooking, with arthritis.
- Learn the use of assistive devices and tools in accomplishing activities of daily living, such as shoe horns for putting on shoes and special utensils for dining.
- Assess safety concerns around the home, such as stairs or rugs that could pose a fall risk.

What is the role of hand therapy in rheumatoid arthritis?

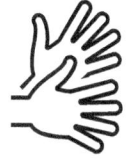

- Improve strength of the fingers and hands.
- Improve dexterity and fine motor control of the hands.
- Decrease pain and improve functionality of the hands.

Examples of Hand Exercises:

- Wrap a rubber band around your fingers. Open and close your fingers, using the rubber band as a resistance band. This increases the strength of the interdigital muscles.
- Touch your tip of your thumb to the tip of the index finger, then the middle finger, ring finger, and pinky finger sequentially. Make a fist with your hand and then stretch the hand into an open palm. Stretch and massage each finger by pulling on it gently. Repeat.
- Get play-doh or a stress ball. Massage the play-doh or stress ball to help with hand strength and to decrease joint stiffness throughout the day.

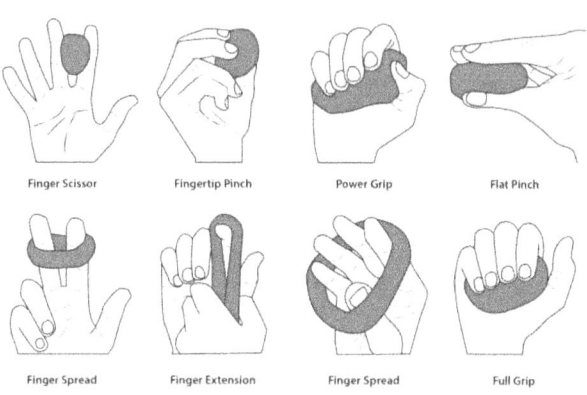

JOINT SURGERY

When should I be referred to an orthopedic surgeon?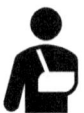

Surgery is meant to be a last resort after all other options are considered and explored. Usually, the minimally invasive strategies such as medications, joint injections, and physical therapy are exhausted before surgery is discussed. Joint surgeries are performed more on patients with generalized osteoarthritis and/or joint injuries rather than for rheumatoid arthritis.

When does rheumatoid arthritis usually require surgery to be done?

In a small number of cases, surgery could be needed for rheumatoid arthritis. I have had a couple of patients with long-standing rheumatoid arthritis since the 1970s who ended up having joint replacements of the metacarpal (knuckle) joints of the hands.

What are the most common joint surgeries that are performed?

- Total knee replacement surgery, meniscus, or ACL procedures.
- Total hip replacement surgery.
- Neck and lower back surgeries for degenerative disc disease and herniated discs.
- Shoulder surgery for rotator cuff issues and shoulder replacement.
- Carpal tunnel surgery.
- Foot surgery for bunions or hammer toes.

What is the difference between an arthroscopic surgery and a total joint replacement surgery?

An arthroscopy is a minimally invasive procedure done with small cameras inserted into joints. Arthroscopic surgery is usually for meniscus tears of the knees and other issues that are relatively easy to fix. A total joint replacement has been done when osteoarthritis has progressed to a severe degree.

Do I have to pause my rheumatoid arthritis medications before I get a surgery done?

Research shows that DMARD medications such as methotrexate, leflunomide, sulfasalazine, and hydroxychloroquine do <u>not</u> have to be stopped before a surgery. Studies show that these DMARD mediations do <u>not</u> pose an increased risk of infection after surgery or delayed healing.

On the other hand, medications such as biologics and JAK inhibitors do have to be stopped 1-2 weeks prior to surgery and are restarted 1-2 weeks after surgery is completed. There can be an increased risk of post-operative infection with biologics and JAK inhibitors.

ASSISTIVE AIDS FOR DAILY LIVING

What are arthritis compression gloves?

Arthritis compression gloves can be worn at night to reduce joint pain, swelling, and morning joint stiffness. Morning joint stiffness occurs because fluid builds up overnight in the hand joints when we don't move as much. When we wake up in the morning, it can take an hour or longer for the fluid to be worked out of the hand joints until they feel better. Wearing compression gloves prevents fluid buildup in the joints overnight as we sleep, which helps with joint pain and reduces the duration of morning joint stiffness.

What can I do for carpal tunnel syndrome?

Carpal tunnel syndrome occurs more frequently in patients with rheumatoid arthritis than the general population because of increased inflammation and arthritic changes in the wrist joints, leading to compression of the median nerve. Symptoms of carpal tunnel syndrome include numbness and tingling of the fingertips, loss of strength in the muscles of the hands, and reduced manual dexterity. Symptoms are usually the worst at night but can occur anytime during the day.

The first step after carpal tunnel syndrome is usually to wear wrist braces at night. Steroid injections can also be given into the wrist joints to reduce inflammation. If those measures don't help, or if there is muscle atrophy of the hands, a hand surgeon will usually offer a carpal tunnel release surgery.

When are orthotic shoes most helpful?

Our feet bear the brunt of our body weight as we walk and stand throughout our lives. Rheumatoid arthritis affects the small joints of the feet, but our feet develop plenty of osteoarthritis throughout our lives as well. Take care of your feet by wearing shoes with good arch support. Avoid wearing flip flops and shoes with no arch support as much as you can!

There are special orthotic shoes that can be tailored to your feet. These can be especially helpful if you have flat feet (the medical term for this is "pes planus"). Flat feet with a low arch can predispose to foot osteoarthritis as well as contribute to abnormal biomechanics of the knees and hips when you walk.

What are other assistive aids for mobility?

- Knee or ankle braces
- A cane for walking
- Walker
- Wheelchair
- Motorized scooter or wheelchair

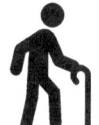

Case scenarios

These case scenarios are illustrations of journeys that different patients may experience, which are loosely based on the paths that some of my patients have taken with physical therapy and surgeries. Names have been changed for anonymity.

Case 1

Charles feels like his hand muscles are becoming weaker from rheumatoid arthritis over time. He is losing grip strength in his fingers, has trouble opening jars and lids, and often drops objects like his coffee cup or keys. He is wondering if there is anything else he can do to prevent his hands from deteriorating, in addition to taking his rheumatoid arthritis medications.

His rheumatologist referred him to a physical therapist specializing in hand therapy. He goes twice a week to the hand therapist to work on hand exercise to strengthen his hand muscles and improve the dexterity of his fingers. He feels that the therapy was helpful and continues to do the exercises on his own at home after the sessions have concluded.

Case 2

Jennifer has knee osteoarthritis in addition to seropositive rheumatoid arthritis. Sometimes it can be difficult to tell which of her joint symptoms are from osteoarthritis and which ones are from rheumatoid arthritis. Her rheumatologist ordered knee x-rays which showed she had severe "bone on bone" osteoarthritis.

Jennifer was referred to an orthopedic surgeon who said that she could delay surgery for a while with knee injections and physical therapy, but eventually she would probably need a total knee replacement surgery when she feels ready. Jennifer needed to use a cane for walking and ended up deciding to get the knee replacement surgery done after about a year or so. She had a smooth recovery from the surgery, and was able to get back to water aerobics and gardening afterwards.

Case 3

Rick had improvement in joint pain and swelling after his rheumatoid arthritis was treated by his rheumatologist. However, within the past couple of months, he has noticed numbness and tingling developing in both hands and in the fingertips. These symptoms wake him up at night and are especially problematic because he owns a mechanic shop and hasn't been able to do detailed work with his hands as easily as before. He often has to stop to shake his hands out because they feel numb.

His rheumatologist suspected carpal tunnel syndrome and a nerve conduction study confirmed the diagnosis. Rick started wearing wrist braces at night, but they weren't helping enough and it was uncomfortable wearing them while he was trying to sleep. He was eventually referred to a hand surgeon who explained that he would probably need a carpal tunnel surgery to fix the problem.

Action list:

- [ ] Find one form of exercise that might be a good fit for you.
- [ ] Start a 5-minute stretching routine every morning when you wake up and every evening before bed.
- [ ] Try the arthritis compression gloves at night when you're sleeping to see if they help with symptoms of morning joint stiffness and pain.

Reflection questions:

1. Have you mostly had positive or negative experiences with exercise? What form of exercise would be more "fun" or enjoyable?

2. Other than joint pain and fatigue, what else might be hindering you from increasing your exercise and activity level?

3. Do you ever get confused about which joint pain symptoms are caused by osteoarthritis versus rheumatoid arthritis? If so, discuss this with your rheumatologist at the next visit.

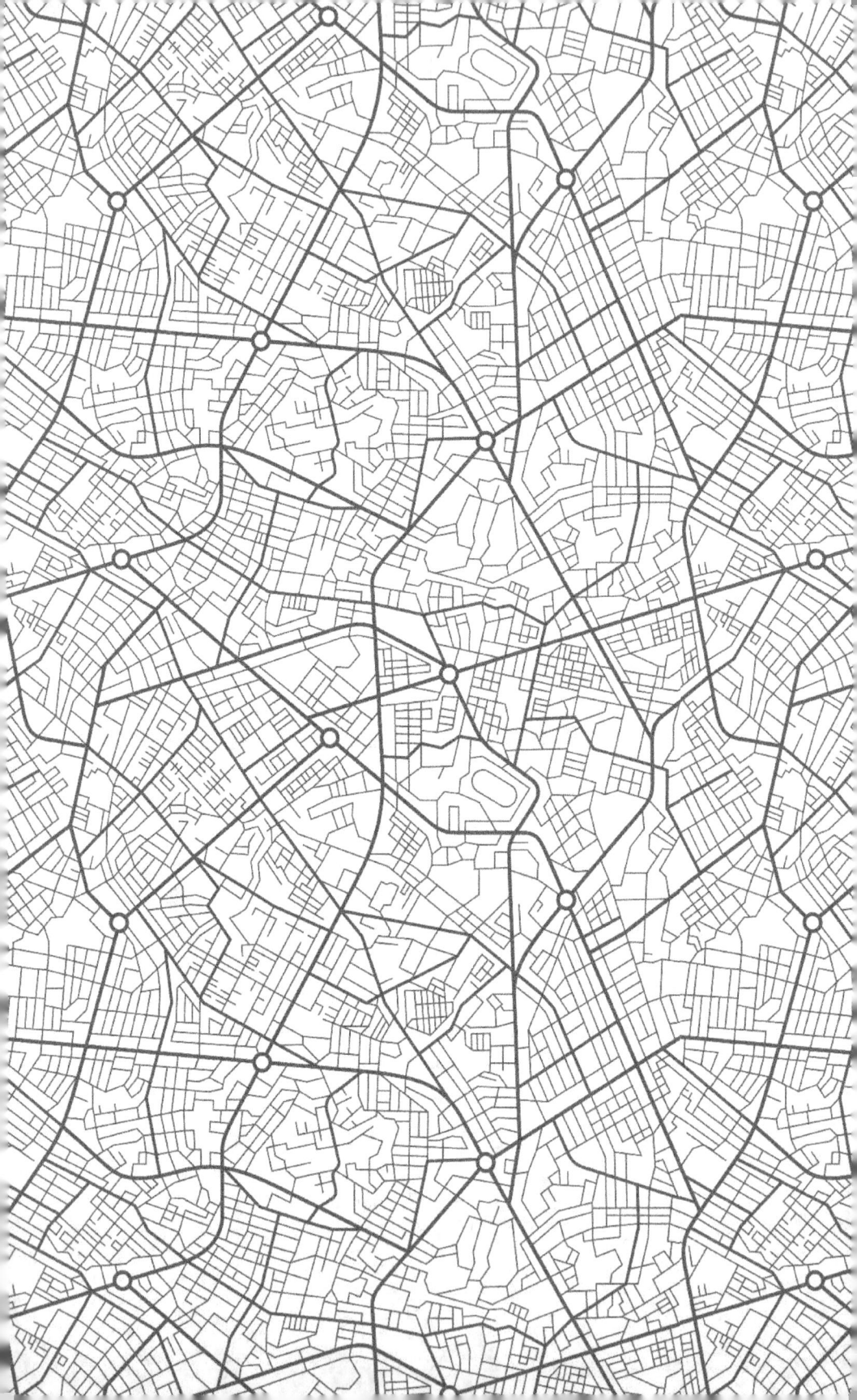

CHAPTER 9

NAVIGATING RHEUMATOID ARTHRITIS DURING THE COVID-19 PANDEMIC

AN UNPRECEDENTED TIME TO BE IMMUNOSUPPRESSED

Am I considered immunosuppressed because I have a diagnosis of rheumatoid arthritis?

Patients with rheumatoid arthritis are considered immunosuppressed for a few reasons:

- The immune system is "distracted" because it is busy with the autoimmune process of attacking its own body, rather than making a concerted effort towards foreign invaders such as bacteria and viruses.
- The medications used to treat inflammation and autoimmune disease cause immunosuppression. This includes steroids, DMARDs, biologics, JAK inhibitors, and the other medications we discussed.
- Patients may not respond as well to vaccines due to taking immunosuppressive medications. This is going to be discussed in further detail in a subsequent section.

Can the COVID-19 vaccine cause or trigger autoimmune diseases like rheumatoid arthritis?

This is a controversial topic that is still being studied. There have been a few case reports of vaccines such as the flu shot triggering symptoms of polymyalgia rheumatica (a painful condition in elderly patients) or other inflammatory conditions. The mechanism behind this is unclear, and it's unknown whether the COVID-19 vaccine has a proven record of directly causing autoimmune diseases such as rheumatoid arthritis and other ones. Some patients have mentioned that they have joint pain and muscle ache symptoms for 24-48 hours after the COVID-19 vaccine which were temporary and resolved without any intervention.

It is going to be difficult to design a research study to differentiate between patients who developed autoimmune disease as a direct result of the vaccines, and those who developed their disease naturally or from a separate process. Time may be able to give us more insights into such mysteries, or it's possible that some relationships may never be proven to exist.

What can I do to decrease my risk of contracting the COVID-19 virus?

The main things that immunosuppressed patients can do to protect themselves against the COVID-19 infection are the same things that anyone else can do:

- Wear a mask around others in public.
- Wash and sanitize hands and surfaces regularly.
- Don't touch your face, nose, and mouth with unwashed hands.
- Get the vaccinations and booster shots done.
- Avoid people who are sick with COVID.
- Avoid crowded areas.
- Consider receiving Evusheld as a preexposure prophylaxis against COVID-19, discussed in more detail below.

Should I get the COVID-19 vaccine?

Yes, it is generally recommended that everyone get vaccinated, but this is especially important for patients who are immunosuppressed. The main reasons not to get the vaccine are allergy or anaphylactic reaction to a prior injection. Vaccines were already controversial before the pandemic started, and they are even more controversial and politicized nowadays! There may be personal or religious reasons why some people wish to avoid vaccinations, and it is each individual's own choice whether or not to receive the vaccine.

Which of the vaccines should I receive? Is there a big difference between the Pfizer, Moderna, and Johnson & Johnson vaccines?

My infectious disease colleagues are mostly recommending the Pfizer or Moderna vaccines for patients who are immunosuppressed. The Pfizer and Moderna vaccines were researched more for patients with underlying conditions and serious comorbidities, while the Johnson & Johnson vaccine was studied more in the young and healthy population.

How do the vaccines work?

All three of the vaccines—from Pfizer, Moderna, and Johnson & Johnson—are mRNA vaccines. Instead of containing antigens and cell pieces from the virus itself like the flu shot does, these COVID vaccines contain the message that the immune system needs to mount a response against the virus without being introduced to any fragment of the virus directly.

Should I get the booster shot (a third dose)?

Yes, it is advisable for patients who are immunosuppressed to receive a booster shot. Most of my patients have already received the booster shot and I have received it as well.

Should I get *another* booster shot (a *fourth* dose)?

By now, we're all wondering exactly how many doses we will be receiving in the end! We are all feeling like pin cushions being stuck over and over again by injections. There is discussion of a 4th shot by summer of 2022 for immunosuppressed patients (if it hasn't been announced already). It's also possible that the COVID booster will be combined with the flu shot into one injection, and we may be receiving it annually every fall or winter.

Is there any benefit of mixing vaccines from different manufacturers for better coverage of variants?

There is debate over whether mixing vaccines from Pfizer and Moderna, or getting further booster shots from different manufacturers has any benefit in covering COVID variants. Overall, getting all of the vaccines and booster doses done is more important than which manufacturer you pick from.

Should I stay away from people who are unvaccinated?

This is another controversial topic that I won't be able to answer clearly with a blanket statement for everyone. Some patients ask me whether they should stop seeing their grandson or granddaughter for a while because they go to daycare and aren't vaccinated. There are too many personal factors in those scenarios and the decision is deeply personal.

I can share what some of my patients have been doing. Some are still seeing family members and friends who aren't vaccinated, but being careful with keeping a mask on and avoiding crowded areas when they meet. Some people are avoiding unvaccinated family and friends entirely and doing more Zoom and virtual hangouts. Some patients who are extra cautious are asking family members to do a nasal swab prior to family gatherings or after traveling to make sure they test negative being seeing them.

Do immunosuppressant medications blunt my immune system's response to vaccinations?

Previous research studies show that DMARD medications such as methotrexate do blunt the immune system's response to vaccines like the flu shot. We haven't had enough time or experience to know exactly how the medications for RA influence the body's response to the COVID-19 vaccine. There haven't been any dedicated research trials, only anecdotal evidence or case reports.

Based on the little data we have so far since 2021 when the vaccines were widely distributed, it seems that a patient's response to the vaccines and booster shots can be diminished from taking RA therapies. However, it's difficult to predict who will be affected and how much. In the majority of my patients taking RA medications, they have still developed the IgG antibodies (the immune system's long-term imprint) against COVID when their labs were checked.

The good news is that most of my patients have had very mild cases of COVID infection despite taking immunosuppressant medications—mostly fatigue and a "head cold" or sinus symptoms in many cases. They recovered normally from COVID infection and didn't have lingering symptoms.

Which of the immunosuppressive medications for RA has the greatest impact on a person's responsiveness to vaccinations?

Patients receiving rituximab infusions seem to have poor response to the vaccines and booster shots, depending on the timing. This is because rituximab directly blocks B-cell activity, which is responsible for producing antibodies for long-term immune memory.

I remember that one of my patients received the rituximab infusion in the hospital right after receiving their second dose of the vaccine. When we tested for COVID IgG antibodies on her several weeks later, they were undetectable. I advised her to repeat the vaccines and she did. The second time around, she did have the COVID IgG antibodies, which was more reassuring.

Should I pause my rheumatoid arthritis medications when receiving the vaccine or booster shot?

You can pause your medications for a few days prior to the vaccine or booster shot and restart the medications a week later. It's unclear how much of a benefit this is doing though, because most medications stay in your system for a while even after stopping them. For example, methotrexate has a half-life of about 2 weeks, so even if you pause it for a while, the medication is still in your system when you receive the shot.

Experts are divided on this topic and say that immunosuppressive medications for RA don't need to be stopped prior to receiving the vaccines or booster shots. No research studies have been done on this subject to determine the best course of action. Patients tend to report that their arthritis flares if they stop their medications for too long, so many of them have continued their medications through the vaccinations.

How useful is it to check for COVID-19 IgG antibodies on lab work?

IgG antibodies are the immune system's long-term memory or imprint for infectious diseases. Once your immune system has developed IgG antibodies against a certain virus, there is a good chance it will mount a quick and adequate response to that foreign invader when exposed again in the future. It is reasonable to ask your primary care provider or rheumatologist to check for IgG antibodies if you are immunosuppressed and want to know if you have adequate protection against COVID or not.

Notably, IgG antibodies cannot distinguish between a previous natural infection to COVID or a response from the vaccine. Thus, if you've been vaccinated already, and are wondering if you've had the actual infection or not in the past, it will be impossible to differentiate between the two.

Should I pause my rheumatoid arthritis medications if I get infected with COVID?

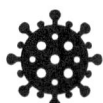

The rule is typically that if you are sick and have a fever and/or are requiring antibiotics, it is best to pause your RA medications until symptoms resolve and antibiotic course is completed. If you are sick with COVID infection, pause your RA medications until your symptoms resolve.

What is post-COVID syndrome?

Patients have reported lingering symptoms after recovering from the initial symptoms of COVID-19 infection. The most frequent symptom in the long haul is fatigue. Shortness of breath, a lingering cough, or phlegm production can also be part of post-COVID syndrome. These symptoms can hang on for several months after the infection.

What are the monoclonal antibody infusions?

The monoclonal antibody infusions are meant for people who have contracted the COVID-19 infection within the past 48 hours and are in the immunosuppressed population. Regeneron, also called bamlanivumab, is one such infusion.

Most infusions have been in short supply around the nation since the surge of the Omicron variant. Receiving the infusion in the first couple days after you test positive for COVID can help you recover much faster and prevent serious hospitalization. It has to be given within a certain time frame.

What is Paxlovid?

Also known as nirmatrelvir-ritonavir, Paxlovid is taken by mouth and works by decreasing COVID viral replication in the body. Paxlovid is still considered investigational, but the FDA authorized this medication for emergency use during the pandemic. It is usually given for immunosuppressed individuals or those who are at high risk for developing complications from COVID-19 infection.

It can only be given to those with mild to moderate symptoms, not patients in the hospital or with severe symptoms from COVID infection. Paxlovid hasn't been studied in pregnancy or for children under the age of 12 yet (as of July 2022). Possible side effects are a metallic taste in the mouth, diarrhea, and a "rebound" effect" with worsening symptoms after the treatment is completed.

Is there anything I can do beyond wearing a mask and washing my hands to protect myself against COVID-19? What is Evusheld?

Evusheld is a new pre-exposure prophylaxis against the COVID-19 infection. This means that even before you are exposed to the virus or become infected, you could provide a protection for yourself if you're in the immunosuppressed population.

This prophylaxis is especially valuable for patients who weren't able to receive all of the vaccines or booster shots due to allergic reactions or other serious side effects. Evusheld is also helpful for patients who were taking immunosuppressive medications when they received the vaccines and may not have had a full immune response to the vaccines. Rheumatoid arthritis patients taking immunosuppressive medications fall into this category.

Case scenarios

These case scenarios are illustrations of journeys that different patients may experience, which are loosely based on the paths that some of my patients have taken with navigating immunosuppression and vaccinations during the COVID-19 pandemic. Names have been changed for anonymity.

Case 1

Matt doesn't usually get any vaccinations, not even the flu shot during fall and winter seasons. When the COVID-19 vaccines came out, he was very reluctant to get vaccinated because it seemed like the vaccines were fast-tracked and had side effects. He wasn't sure what an "mRNA vaccine" meant and whether it would have long-term effects on his immune system.

Since Matt is taking immunosuppressive medications for his rheumatoid arthritis, he was worried about contracting a serious illness due to COVID and becoming one of the hospitalized and intubated patients he saw on the news. He decided to go ahead and get the vaccine done. He had a flare of joint pain that lasted about a day after getting the first dose of the vaccine, but no other major issues. He went on to receive the second dose and the booster shot.

Case 2

Phyllis received her rituximab infusion for rheumatoid arthritis about one week after receiving the second dose of the COVID-19 vaccine. Out of curiosity, we checked for COVID IgG antibodies to see if her immune system produced them. We found out she had undetectable levels of antibodies against COVID on her lab work.

She received the vaccines again, and this time around, we made sure to schedule her rituximab infusions about one month after the second dose in order to give her immune system an adequate chance to respond to the vaccines. Upon rechecking her labs again later, Phyllis was found to have the IgG antibodies against COVID.

Case 3

Abigail is taking three medications for rheumatoid arthritis. She has also had asthma since childhood and has severe anxiety about the pandemic and getting seriously sick or hospitalized with COVID-19 infection. The anxiety has been crippling and she has been avoiding all social situations and has mostly been home bound since the beginning of 2020.

However, Abigail is getting married in 3 months and will be around family and friends for the first time in a couple of years. A lot of her family and friends aren't vaccinated and many of them don't like wearing masks either. After discussion with her rheumatologist about her fears, they decided that Abigail is a candidate for receiving Evusheld and she is going to go ahead and get it done before her wedding day to give herself pre-exposure protection against COVID infection.

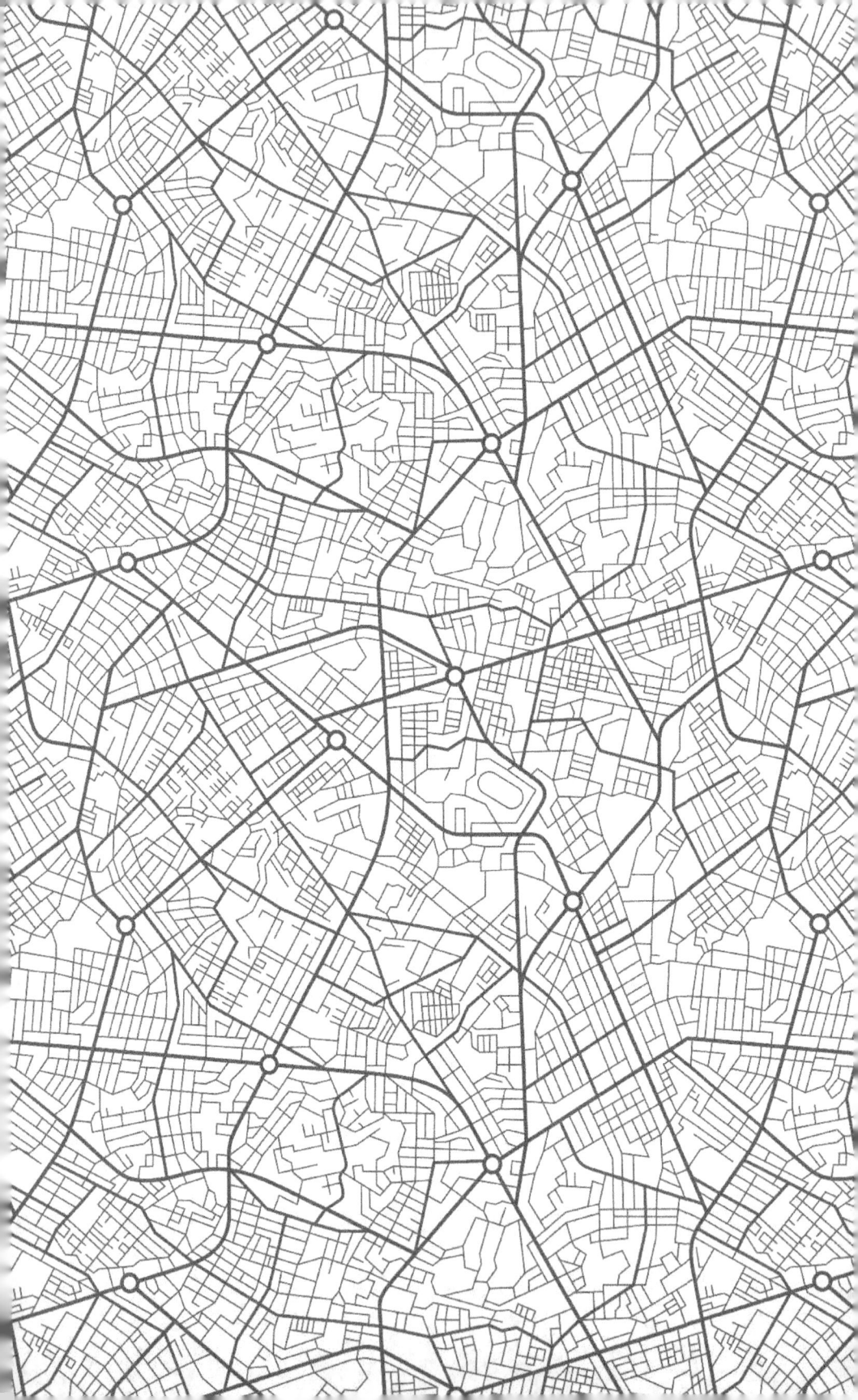

CHAPTER 10
PUTTING IT ALL TOGETHER

YOUR PERSONAL JOURNEY WITH RHEUMATOID ARTHRITIS

"There are no drugs to treat suffering. But giving meaning to an illness through the creation of a story is one way in which suffering can be relieved." [Eric Cassell]

By now, you've seen that the journeys through rheumatoid arthritis are widely variable and can be extremely different for each individual. You may have taken a completely different route to arrive at  your diagnosis than someone else did. Your preferences for treatment may be vastly different than another person's. You can individualize and tailor your treatment plan based on what you and your rheumatologist decide together. Health and healing are unique to each individual and may differ for two people with the same disease.

Your individual journey could be anywhere on a spectrum, including the following:

- ❖ Conventional Western medicine treatments such as DMARDs, biologics, JAK inhibitors, or a combination of any of these prescription medications.
- ❖ A primarily holistic and alternative approach with the anti-inflammatory diet, vitamins, supplements, exercise, and other lifestyle changes.
- ❖ A focus on minimally invasive strategies for chronic pain such as physical therapy and steroid injections into affected joints.'
- ❖ An early surgical approach to maximize quality of life such as joint replacement or spine surgery to relieve pain when other treatments have failed.

In thinking about your health and personal goals for the future, it is helpful to identify what being "healthy" really means to you. For some, "health" might look like being able to keep up with their grandkids and being able to play with them. For others, being "healthy" might mean running three marathons per year or achieving their lifelong dream of climbing Mount Everest.

What gives your life a sense of meaning and purpose? If you were healthy, what would your life look like? Why do you want to be healthy or improve your health? Identify your individual and specific health goals for the next few years and write them here:

_____

_____

_____

_____

_____

The journey of health begins with ourselves, is supported by those around us such as family, friends, community, and healthcare professionals, is influenced by our lifestyle choices, and is shaped by our inner and outer environments.

Think about next steps in achieving your health goals. Where do you need to start the healing process? What are one or two areas that you feel you need to work on most to achieve your goals? Who do you need to support you in achieving your health goals? Write it down here:

_____

_____

_____
_____
_____
_____
_____
_____
_____
_____
_____
_____

In achieving your goals and having the right mindset to accomplish them, it is helpful to focus your mind on the right thought processes. I recently read a wonderful book called "7 Thoughts to Live Your Life By," written by I.C. Robledo. It has changed my life and I highly recommend it to everyone.

Here, I will quote the author and include a bit about the 7 Thoughts that he writes about:

1. "Focus on what you can control, not on what you can't control.
2. Focus on what you have, not what you don't have.
3. Focus on what you can do, not what you can't do.
4. Focus on the positive, not the negative.
5. Focus on the present, not the past or future.

6. Focus on what you need, not what you want.
7. Focus on what you can give, not what you can take or receive."

I believe these concepts can be applied to any life scenario, including living with rheumatoid arthritis. Here are some ways to think about your rheumatoid arthritis diagnosis to stay inspired and encouraged despite having a painful condition.

1. **Focus on what you can control, not on what you can't control.** "I didn't have any control over being diagnosed with rheumatoid arthritis, but I do have control over my treatments and can focus on how to feel better and prevent my joints from becoming damaged."

2. **Focus on what you have, not what you don't have.** "These immunosuppressive medications sound scary, but at least we do have effective treatments for rheumatoid arthritis nowadays as opposed to no treatment options in the past."

3. **Focus on what you can do, not what you can't do.** "I can't do gardening all day like I used to love to do, but I can still garden in short spurts and find new hobbies that I enjoy doing."

4. **Focus on the positive, not the negative.** "I'm not living completely pain-free, but over time I am having fewer and fewer flares of joint pain as my treatments are kicking in. I always wanted to eat healthier and live a healthier lifestyle, and now my arthritis is compelling me to do that instead of waiting."

5. **Focus on the present, not the past or future.** "I'm worried about what my joints will be like in 20 to 30 years, and whether I'll be functional or not, but I'm going to choose to live today the best way I can, even with my arthritis."

6. **Focus on what you need, not what you want.** "What I really want or wish is for my rheumatoid arthritis to go away completely and not have to take medications to feel better, but what I need is to reach remission so I can live an active lifestyle, work as long as I want to, and be there for my family. I know I can achieve that, given time."

7. **Focus on what you can give, not what you can take or receive.** "I can still give back to my community with rheumatoid arthritis, and it has helped me understand what other people with chronic pain and illness go through. I can use my empathy and new perspectives for a greater good."

No matter where you are in processing your diagnosis and condition, I wish you the absolute best on your integrative journey to health and wellness. I believe you can still live your best life, full of joy and peace, despite your arthritis, as I have seen many of my patients get to do!

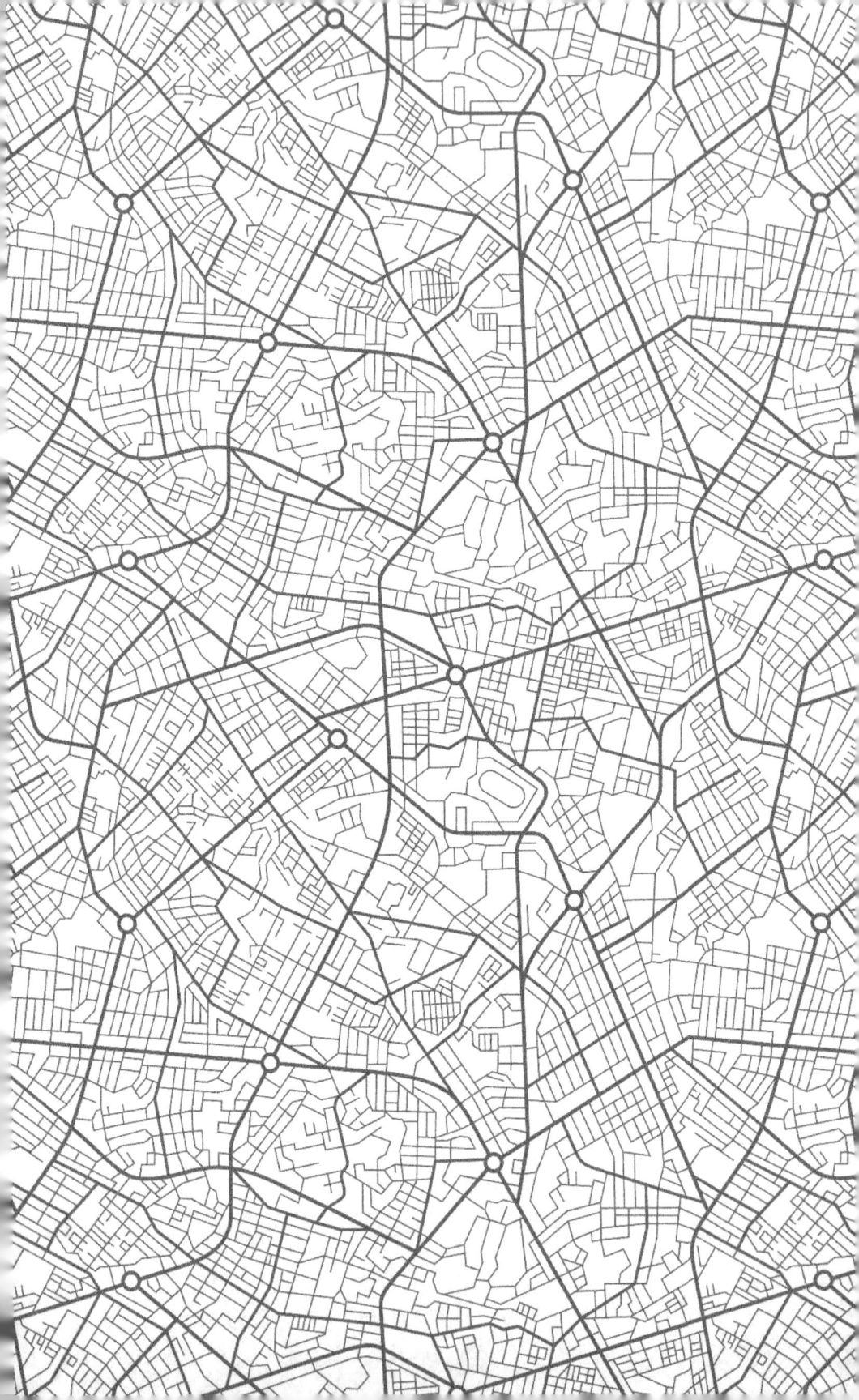

DISCLAIMER

The information given in this book is not intended to replace the advice given to you by your health care providers and professionals. If you have any concerns about your health, contact your rheumatologist or health professional. The author disclaims any liability directly or indirectly from the use of the material in this book by any person.

The names of all individuals mentioned in this book have been changed or disguised to protect their privacy.

ADDITIONAL RESOURCES

Recommended reading:

- "The Complete Anti-inflammatory Diet for Beginners" by Dorothy Calimeris and Lulu Cook
- "The Anti-inflammatory Diet Cookbook" by Madeline Given and Jennifer Lang
- "The Body Keeps the Score: Brain, Mind, and Body in the Healing of Trauma" by Dr. Bessel Van Der Kolk
- "Stretching to Stay Young" by Jessica Matthews
- "7 Thoughts to Live Your Life By" by I.C. Robledo
- "Built from Broken: A Science-Based Guide to Healing Painful Joints, Preventing Injuries, and Rebuilding Your Body" by Scott Hogan
- "Boundless Energy: the Complete Mind/Body Program for Overcoming Chronic Fatigue" by Deepak Chopra

- ❖ "Radiant Rest: Yoga Nidra for Deep Relaxation and Awakened Clarity" by Tracee Stanley
- ❖ "Yoga for Arthritis: The Complete Guide" by Loren Fishman and Ellen Saltonstall
- ❖ "Every Patient Tells a Story: Medical Mysteries and the Art of Diagnosis" by Lisa Sanders

Support groups for rheumatoid arthritis:

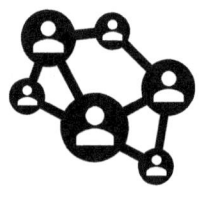

- The Arthritis Foundation
- Rheumatoid Arthritis Healing Naturally Support Group
- Rheumatoid Arthritis Support and Awareness Group
- Squeaky Joints support group

Research and advocacy:

- American College of Rheumatology
- National Center for Complementary and Integrative Health
- Academy of Integrative Health and Medicine
- Arthritis Care & Research

REFERENCES

1. West, Sterling and Kolfenbach, Jason. Rheumatology Secrets. Fourth edition, 2019.

2. Rakel, David. Integrative Medicine. 4th edition, 2018.

3. Bird P., Griffiths H., Tymms K., et al: The Simle study – safety of methotrexate in combination with leflunomide in rheumatoid arthritis. J Rheumatol 2013; 40: pp. 228-235

4. Braun et al., 2008. Braun J., Kastner P., and Flaxenberg P.: Comparison of the clinical efficacy and safety of subcutaneous versus oral administration of methotrexate in patients with active rheumatoid arthritis. Arthritis Rheum 2008; 58: pp. 73-81

5. Cannella and O'Dell, 2017. Cannella A.C., and O'Dell J.R.: Traditional DMARDs: methotrexate, leflunomide, sulfasalazine, hydroxychloroquine, and combination therapies. In Firestein G.S. (eds): Kelley & Firestein's Textbook of Rheumatology, 10th ed. Philadelphia: Elsevier, 2017. pp. 958-982

6. Felson et al., 1995. Felson D.T., Anderson J.J., Boers M., et al: American college of rheumatology preliminary definition for improvement in rheumatoid arthritis. Arthritis Rheum 1995; 38: pp. 727-735

7. Hoekstra et al., 2006. Hoekstra M., Haagsma C., Neef C., et al: Splitting high dose oral methotrexate improves the bioavailability: a pharmacokinetic study in patients with rheumatoid arthritis. J Rheumatol 2006; 33: pp. 481-485

8. Izmirly et al., 2012. Izmirly P.M., Costedoat-Chalumeau N., Bunyon J.P., et al: Maternal use of hydroxychloroquine is associated with a reduced risk of recurrent anti-SSA/Ro antibody–associated cardiac manifestations of neonatal lupus. Circulation 2012; 126: pp. 76-82

9. Katz and Russell, 2011. Katz S.J., and Russell A.S.: Re-evaluation of antimalarials in treating rheumatic diseases: re-appreciation and insights into new mechanisms of action. Curr Opin Rheumatol 2011; 23: pp. 278-281

10. Kremer, 2004. Kremer J.: Toward a better understanding of methotrexate. Arthritis Rheum 2004; 50: pp. 1370-1382

11. Landewe et al., 2002. Landewe R.B.M., Boers M., Verhoeven A.C., et al: COBRA combination therapy in patients with early rheumatoid arthritis: long-term structural benefits of a brief intervention. Arthritis Rheum 2002; 46: pp. 347-356

12. Marmor et al., 2016. Marmor M.F., Kellner U., Lai T.Y., Melles R.B., and Mieler W.F.: Recommendations on screening for chloroquine and hydroxychloroquine retinopathy (2016 Revision). Ophthalmology 2016; 123: pp. 1386-1394

13. Melles and Marmor, 2014. Melles R.B., and Marmor M.F.: The risk of toxic retinopathy in patients on long-term hydroxychloroquine therapy. JAMA Ophthalmol 2014; 132: pp. 1453-1460

14. Moreland et al., 2012. Moreland L.W., O'Dell J.R., Paulus H.E., et al: A randomized comparative effectiveness study of oral triple therapy versus etanercept plus methotrexate in early aggressive rheumatoid arthritis: the treatment of early aggressive rheumatoid arthritis trial. Arthritis Rheum 2012; 64: pp. 2824-2835

15. O'Dell et al., 1996. O'Dell J.R., Haire C., Erikson N., et al: Treatment of rheumatoid arthritis with methotrexate, sulfasalazine, and hydroxychloroquine, or a combination of these medications. N Engl J Med 1996; 334: pp. 1287-1291

16. O'Dell et al., 1997. O'Dell J.R., Haire C.E., Moore G.F., et al: Treatment of early rheumatoid arthritis with minocycline or placebo. Arthritis Rheum 1997; 40: pp. 842-848

17. Plosker and Croom, 2005. Plosker G., and Croom K.: Sulfasalazine: a review of its use in the management of rheumatoid arthritis. Drugs 2005; 65: pp. 1825-1849

18. SinghSaag and Bridges, 2015. Singh J.A., Saag K.G., Bridges S.L., et al: American College of Rheumatology guideline for the treatment of rheumatoid arthritis. Arthritis Care Res 2015; 68: pp. 1-26

19. Smolen et al., 1999. Smolen J., Kalden J.R., Scott D.L., et al: Efficacy and safety of leflunomide compared with placebo and sulphasalazine in active rheumatoid arthritis: a double-blind, randomized, multicentre trial. Lancet 1999; 353: pp. 259-266

20. Smolen et al., 2017. Smolen J.S., Landewe R., Bijlsma J., et al: EULAR recommendations for the management of rheumatoid arthritis with synthetic and biological disease-modifying antirheumatic drugs: 2016 update. Ann Rheum Dis 2017; 76: pp. 960-977

21. Wolfe and Marmor, 2010. Wolfe F., and Marmor M.F.: Rates and predictors of hydroxychloroquine retinal toxicity in patients with rheumatoid arthritis and systemic lupus erythematosus. Arthritis Care Res 2010; 62: pp. 775-784

22. Allem et al., 2019. Allem K.B., and Keating R.M.: Immunosuppressive agents: cyclosporine, cyclophosphamide, azathioprine, mycophenolate mofetil, and tacrolimus. In Hochberg M.C. (eds): Rheumatology, 7th ed. Philadelphia: Elsevier, 2019. pp. 518-526

23. Fields et al., 1998. Fields C.L., Robinson J.W., Roy T.M., et al: Hypersensitivity reaction to azathioprine. South Med J 1998; 91: pp. 471-474

24. Perez et al., 2017. Perez E.E., Orange J.S., Bonilla F., Chinen J., Chinn I.K., Dorsey M., et al: Update on the use of immunoglobulin in human disease: a review of evidence. J Allergy Clin Immunol 2017; 139: pp. S1-S46

25. Schedel et al., 2006. Schedel J., Godde A., Schutz E., et al: Impact of thiopurine methyltransferase activity and 6-thioguanine nucleotide concentrations in

patients with chronic inflammatory diseases. Ann NY Acad Sci 2006; 1069: pp. 477-491

26. Schwartz et al., 2017. Schwartz D.M., Kanno Y., Villarino A., et al: JAK inhibition as a strategy for immune and inflammatory diseases. Nature Rev Drug Discovery 2017; 16: pp. 843-862

27. Smolen et al., 2017. Smolen J.S., Landewe R., Bijlsma J., et al: Eular recommendations for the management of rheumatoid arthritis with synthetic and biological disease-modifying antirheumatic drugs: 2016 update. Ann Rheum Dis 2017; 76: pp. 960-977

28. Vazquez et al., 2008. Vazquez S.R., Rondina M.T., and Pendleton R.C.: Azathioprine-induced warfarin resistance. Ann Pharmacother 2008; 42: pp. 1118-1123

29. Aaltonen et al., 2012. Aaltonen K.J., Virkki L.M., Malmivarra A., et al: Systematic review and meta-analysis of the efficacy and safety of existing TNF blocking agents in treatment of rheumatoid arthritis. PLOS ONE 2012

30. Bredemeir et al., 2014. Bredemeir M., de Oliveira F.K., and Rocha C.M.: Low versus high dose rituximab for rheumatoid arthritis: a systemic review and meta-analysis. Arthritis Care Res 2014; 66: pp. 228-235

31. Campbell et al., 2011. Campbell L., Chen C., Bhagat S.S., et al: Risk of adverse events including serious infections in rheumatoid arthritis patients treated with tocilizumab: a systematic literature review and meta-analysis of randomized controlled trials. Rheumatology 2011; 50: pp. 552-562

32. Chen and Flies, 2013. Chen L., and Flies D.B.: Molecular mechanisms of T cell co-stimulation and co-inhibition. Nat Rev Immunol 2013; 13: pp. 227-242

33. Cohen et al., 2006. Cohen S.B., Emery P., Greenwald M.W., et al: Rituximab for rheumatoid arthritis refractory to anti-tumor necrosis factor therapy: results of a multicenter, randomized, double-blind, placebo-controlled phase III trial evaluating primary efficacy and safety at twenty-four weeks. Arthritis Rheum 2006; 54: pp. 2793-2806

34. Dao and Cush, 2012. Dao K., and Cush J.J.: A vaccination primer for rheumatologists. Drug Safety Quarterly 2012

35. Deepak et al., 2013. Deepak P., Stobaugh D.J., Sherid M., et al: Neurological events with tumour necrosis factor alpha reported to the food and drug administration adverse event reporting system. Aliment Pharmacol Ther 2013; 38: pp. 388-396

36. Dorner and Kay, 2015. Dorner T., and Kay J.: Biosimilars in rheumatology: current perspectives and lessons learnt. Nat Rev Rheumatol 2015; 11: pp. 713-724

37. Engel et al., 2011. Engel P., Gomez Puerta J.A., Ramos Casals M., et al: Therapeutic targeting of B cells for rheumatic autoimmune diseases. Pharmacol Rev 2011; 6: pp. 127-156

38. Flint et al., 2016. Flint J., Panchal S., Hurrell A., et al: BSR and BHPR guideline on prescribing drugs in pregnancy and breastfeeding-Part I: standard and biologic disease modifying anti-rheumatic drugs and corticosteroids. Rheumatology 2016; 55: pp. 1693-1697

39. Genovese et al., 2015. Genovese M.C., Fleischmann R., Kivitz A.J., et al: Sarilumab plus methotrexate in patients with active rheumatoid arthritis and inadequate response to methotrexate: results of a phase III study. Arthritis Rheumatol 2015; 67: pp. 1424-1437

40. Goodman et al., 2017. Goodman S.M., Springer B., Guyatt G., et al: 2017 American College of Rheumatology/ American Association of Hip and Knee Surgeons guideline for the perioperative management of antirheumatic medication in patients with rheumatic diseases undergoing elective total hip or total knee arthroplasty. Arthritis Rheumatol 2017; 69: pp. 1538-1551

41. Joensuu et al., 2015. Joensuu J.T., Huoponen S., Aaltonen K.J., et al: The cost-effectiveness of biologics for the treatment of rheumatoid arthritis: a systemic review. PLoS ONE 2015

42. Kerbleski and Gottlieb, 2009. Kerbleski J.F., and Gottlieb A.B.: Dermatological complications and safety of anti-TNF treatments. Gut 2009; 58: pp. 1033-1039

43. Kremer et al., 2006. Kremer J.M., Genant H.K., Moreland L.W., et al: Effects of abatacept in patients with methotrexate-resistant active rheumatoid arthritis: a randomized trial. Ann Int Med 2006; 144: pp. 865-876

44. Lloyd et al., 2010. Lloyd S., Bujkiewicz S., Wailoo A.J., et al: The effectiveness of anti-TNF-α therapies when used sequentially in rheumatoid arthritis patients: a systematic review and meta-analysis. Rheumatology 2010; 49: pp. 2313-2321

45. Mariette et al., 2011. Mariette X., Matucci-Cerinic M., Pavelka K., et al: Malignancies associated with tumor necrosis factor inhibitors in registries and prospective observational studies: a systematic review and meta-analysis. Ann Rheum Dis 2011; 70: pp. 1895-1904

46. Mastroianni et al., 2011. Mastroianni C.M., Lichtner M., Del Borgo C., et al: Current trends in management of hepatitis B virus reactivation in the biologic therapy era. World J Gastroenterol 2011; 17: pp. 3881-3887

47. Patkar et al., 2008. Patkar N.M., Teng G.G., Curtis J.R., et al: Association of infections and tuberculosis with antitumor necrosis factor alpha therapy. Curr Opin Rheumatol 2008; 20: pp. 320-326

48. Ramos-Casals et al., 2008. Ramos-Casals M., Brito-Zeron P., Munoz S., et al: A systematic review of the off-label use of biological therapies in systemic autoimmune diseases. Medicine 2008; 87: pp. 345-364

49. Rubbert-Roth and Finckh, 2009. Rubbert-Roth A., and Finckh A.: Treatment options in rheumatoid arthritis failing TNF inhibitor therapy: a critical review. Arthritis Res Ther 2009; 11: pp. 51

50. Salliot et al., 2011. Salliot C., Finckh A., Katchamart W., et al: Indirect comparison of the efficacy of biologic antirheumatic agents in rheumatoid

arthritis in patients with an inadequate response to conventional disease-modifying antirheumatic drugs or to an anti-tumor necrosis factor agent: a meta-analysis. Ann Rheum Dis 2011; 70: pp. 266-271

51. Schiff, 2011. Schiff M.: Abatacept treatment for rheumatoid arthritis. Rheumatology 2011; 50: pp. 437-449

52. Singh et al., 2015. Singh J.A., Cameron C., Noorbaloochi S., et al: Risk of serious infection in biological treatment of patients with rheumatoid arthritis: a systemic review and meta-analysis. Lancet 2015; 386: pp. 258-265

53. Singh et al., 2015. Singh J.A., Saag K.G., Bridges S.L., et al: 2015 American College of Rheumatology guideline for the treatment of rheumatoid arthritis. Arthritis Rheumatol 2016; 68: pp. 1-26

54. Smolen et al., 2008. Smolen J.S., Beaulieu A., Rubbert-Roth A., et al: Effect of interleukin 6 receptor inhibition with tocilizumab in patients with rheumatoid arthritis (OPTION study): a double-blind, placebo-controlled randomized trial. Lancet 2008; 371: pp. 987-997

55. Solomon et al., 2013. Solomon D.H., Rassen J.A., Kuriya B., et al: Heart failure risk among patients with rheumatoid arthritis starting a TNF antagonist. Ann Rheum Dis 2013; 72: pp. 1813-1818

56. Tanaka and Kishimoto, 2014. Tanaka T., and Kishimoto T.: The biology and medical implications of interleukin 6. Cancer Immunol Res 2014; 2: pp. 288

57. Tesfa et al., 2011. Tesfa D., Ajeganova S., Hagglund H., et al: Late onset neutropenia following rituximab therapy in rheumatic diseases: association with B lymphocyte depletion and infections. Arthritis Rheumatol 2011; 63: pp. 2209-2214

58. Winthrop et al., 2009. Winthrop K.L., Chang E., Yamashita S., et al: Nontuberculosis mycobacteria infections and anti-tumor necrosis factor α therapy. Emerg Infect Dis 2009; 15: pp. 1556-1561

59. Winthrop et al., 2013. Winthrop K.L., et al: Mycobacterial diseases and antitumor necrosis factor therapy in USA. Ann Rheum Dis 2013; 72: pp. 37-42

60. Choi et al., 2018 5. Choi H., Neogi T., Stamp L., Dalbeth N., and Terkeltaub R.: Implications of the cardiovascular safety of febuxostat and allopurinol in patients with gout and cardiovascular morbidities (CARES) trial and associated FDA public safety alert. Arthritis Rheumatol 2018.

61. Adler et al., 2016. Adler R.A., Fuleihan G.E. H., Bauer D.C., et al: Managing osteoporosis in patients on long-term bisphosphonate treatment: report of a task force of the American Society for Bone and Mineral Research. J Bone Min Res 2016; 31: pp. 16-35

62. Axelsson et al., 2017. Axelsson K.F., Nilsson A.G., Wedel H., et al: Association between alendronate use and hip fracture risk in older patients using oral prednisolone. JAMA 2017; 318: pp. 146-155

63. Bindon et al., 2018. Bindon B., Adams W., Balasubramanian N., et al: Osteoporosis fractures during bisphosphonate drug holidays. Endocrine Pract 2018; 24: pp. 163-169

64. Black and Rosen, 2016. Black D.M., and Rosen C.J.: Postmenopausal osteoporosis. N Engl J Med 2016; 374: pp. 254-262

65. Bonnick et al., 2001. Bonnick S., Johnston C.C., Kleerekoper M., et al: Importance of precision in bone density measurements. J Clin Densitometry 2001; 4: pp. 1-6

66. Buckley et al., 2017. Buckley L., Guyatt G., Fink H.A., et al: 2017 American College of Rheumatology guideline for the prevention and treatment of glucocorticoid-induced osteoporosis. Arthritis Rheum 2017; 69: pp. 1521-1537

67. Camacho et al., 2016. Camacho P.M., Petak S.M., Binkley N., et al: American Association of Clinical Endocrinologists and American College of Endocrinology clinical practice guidelines for the diagnosis and treatment of postmenopausal osteoporosis – 2016. Endocrine Pract 2016; 22: pp. 1-42

68. Crandall et al., 2014. Crandall C.J., Newberry S.J., Diamant A., et al: Comparative effectiveness of pharmacologic treatments to prevent fractures: an updated systematic review. Ann Intern Med 2014; 161: pp. 711-723

69. Cummings et al., 2017. Cummings S.R., Cosman F., Lewiecki E.M., et al: Goal-directed treatment for osteoporosis: a progress report from the ASBMR-NOF working group on goal-directed treatment for osteoporosis. J Bone Min Res 2017; 32: pp. 3-10

70. Dawson-Hughes and Bischoff-Ferrari, 2007. Dawson-Hughes B., and Bischoff-Ferrari H.A.: Therapy of osteoporosis with calcium and vitamin D. J Bone Min Res 2007; 22: pp. V59-63

71. Holick, 2007. Holick M.F.: Vitamin D deficiency. N Engl J Med 2007; 357: pp. 266-281

72. Rothman et al., 2017. Rothman M.S., Lewiecki E.M., and Miller P.D.: Bone density testing is the best way to monitor osteoporosis. Am J Med 2017; 130: pp. 1133-1134

73. Buttgereit et al., 2013. Buttgereit F., Mehta D., Kirwan J., et al: Low-dose prednisone chronotherapy for rheumatoid arthritis: a randomized clinical trial (CAPRA-2). Ann Rheum Dis 2013; 72: pp. 204-210

74. Curtis et al., 2006. Curtis J.R., Westfall A.O., Allison J., et al: Population-based assessment of adverse events associated with long-term glucocorticoid use. Arthritis Rheum 2006; 55: pp. 420-426

75. Hench et al., 1949. Hench P.S., Kendall E.C., Slocumb C.H., et al: The effect of a hormone of the adrenal cortex (17 hydroxy-11-dehydrocorticosterone: compound E) and of pituitary adrenocorticotropic hormone on rheumatoid arthritis: preliminary report. Proc Staff Meet Mayo Clin 1949; 24: pp. 181-197

76. Richter et al., 2002. Richter B., Neises G., and Clar C.: Glucocorticoid withdrawal schemes in chronic medical disorders. A systemic review. Endocrinol Metab Clin North Am 2002; 31: pp. 751-778

77. Saag and Buttgereit, 2019. Saag K., and Buttgereit F.: Systemic glucocorticoid therapy in rheumatology. In Hochberg M.C. (eds): Rheumatology, 7th ed. Philadelphia: Elsevier, 2019. pp. 488-498

78. Stahn and Buttgereit, 2008. Stahn C., and Buttgereit F.: Genomic and nongenomic effects of glucocorticoids. Nat Clin Pract Rheumatol 2008; 4: pp. 525-533

79. Strehl et al., 2016. Strehl C., Bijlsma J.W., de Wit M., et al: Defining conditions where long term glucocorticoid treatment has an acceptably low level of harm to facilitate implementation of existing recommendations: viewpoints from an EULAR task force. Ann Rheum Dis 2016; 75: pp. 952-957

80. Waljee et al., 2017. Waljee A.K., Rogers M.A., Lin P., et al: Short term use of oral corticosteroids and related harms among adults in the United States: population based cohort study. BMJ 2017; 357: pp. 1415

81. Bally and Dendukuri, 2017 9. Bally M., and Dendukuri N.: Risk of acute myocardial infarction with NSAIDs in real world use: bayesian meta-analysis of individual patient data. BMJ 2017; 357: pp. 1909

82. Bhala N (on behalf of NSAID Trialists Collaboration), 2013. Vascular and upper gastrointestinal effects of non-steroidal anti-inflammatory drugs: meta-analyses of individual participant data from randomized trials. Lancet 2013; 382: pp. 769-779

83. Capone et al., 2005. Capone M.L., Sciulli M.G., Tacconelli S., et al: Pharmacodynamic interaction of naproxen with low-dose aspirin in healthy subjects. J. Am. Coll. Cardiol. 2005; 45: pp. 1295-1301

84. Castelli and Petrone, 2017. Castelli G., and Petrone A.: Rates of nonsteroidal anti-inflammatory drug use in patients with established cardiovascular disease: a retrospective, cross-sectional study from NHANES 2009-2010. Am J Cardiovasc Drugs 2017 Jun; 17: pp. 243-249

85. Catella-Lawson et al., 2001. Catella-Lawson F., Reilly M.P., Kapoor S.C., et al: Cyclooxygenase inhibitors and the antiplatelet effects of aspirin. N Engl J Med 2001; 345: pp. 1809-1817

86. Chan et al., 2001. Chan F.K., Chung S.C., Suen B.Y., et al: Preventing recurrent upper gastrointestinal bleeding in patients with Helicobacter pylori infection who are taking low-dose aspirin or naproxen. N Engl J Med 2001; 344: pp. 967-973

87. Chan et al., 2004. Chan F.K., Hung L.C., Suen B.Y., et al: Celecoxib versus diclofenac plus omeprazole in high risk patients: results of a randomized double-blind trial. Gastroenterology 2004; 127: pp. 1038-1043

88. Chan et al., 2007. Chan F.K., Wong V.W., Suen B.Y., et al: Combination of a COX-2 inhibitor and a proton pump inhibitor for the prevention of recurrent

ulcer bleeding in patients at very high risk: a double blind, randomized trial. Lancet 2007; 369: pp. 1621-1626

89. Davis and Lee, 2017. Davis J.S., and Lee H.Y.: Use of non-steroidal anti-inflammatory drugs in US adults: changes over time and by demographic. Open Heart 2017

90. Garcia Rodriquez et al., 2008. Garcia Rodriquez L.A., Tacconelli S., and Patrignani P.: Role of dose potency in the prediction of risk of myocardial infarction associated with nonsteroidal anti-inflammatory drugs in the general population. J Am Coll Cardiol 2008; 52: pp. 1628-1636

91. Lanas, 2005. Lanas A.: Gastrointestinal injury from NSAID therapy: how to reduce the risk of complications. Postgrad Med 2005; 117: pp. 13

92. Lanza et al., 2009. Lanza F.L., Chan F.K., and Quigley E.M.: Guidelines for prevention of NSAID-related ulcer complications. Am J Gastroenter 2009; 104: pp. 728-738

93. McAdam et al., 1999. McAdam B.F., Catella-Lawson F., Mardini I.A., et al: Systemic biosynthesis of prostacyclin by COX-2: the human pharmacology of a selective inhibitor of COX-2. Proc Natl Acad Sci USA 1999; 96: pp. 272-277

94. Nissen and Yeomans, 2016. Nissen S.E., and Yeomans N.D.: Cardiovascular safety of celecoxib, naproxen, or ibuprofen for arthritis. N Engl J Med 2016; 375: pp. 2519-2529

95. Schjerning et al., 2011. Schjerning O.A.M., Fosbøl E.L., Lindhardsen J., et al: Duration of treatment with NSAIDs and impact on risk of death and recurrent myocardial infarction in patients with prior myocardial infarction: a nationwide cohort study. Circulation 2011; 123: pp. 2226-2235

96. Zhou and Freedman, 2014. Zhou Y., and Freedman A.N.: Trends in the use of aspirin and nonsteroidal anti-inflammatory drugs in the general U.S. population. Pharmacoepidemiol Drug Saf 2014 Jan; 23: pp. 43-50

97. Izmirly et al., 2012. Izmirly P.A., Costedoat-Chalumeau N., Pisoni C.N., et al: Maternal use of hydroxychloroquine is associated with a reduced risk of recurrent SSA associated cardiac manifestations of neonatal lupus syndrome. Circulation 2012; 126: pp. 76-82

98. Marder et al., 2016. Marder W., Littlejohn E.A., and Somers E.C.: Pregnancy and autoimmune connective tissue diseases. Best Pract Res Clin Rheumatol 2016; 30: pp. 63-80

99. Østensen et al., 2012. Østensen M., Villiger P.M., and Förger F.: Interaction of pregnancy and autoimmune rheumatic disease. Autoimmun Rev 2012; 11: pp. A437-A446

100. Sammaritano, 2017. Sammaritano L.R.: Contraception in patients with rheumatic disease. Rheum Dis Clin North Am 2017; 43: pp. 173-188

101. Van den Brandt et al., 2017. van den Brandt S., Zbinden A., Baeten D., Villiger P.M., Ostensen M., and Forger F.: Risk factors for flare and treatment of disease flares during pregnancy in rheumatoid arthritis and axial spondyloarthritis patients. *Arthritis Res Ther* 2017; 19: pp. 64

102. D.M. Eisenberg, R.C. Kessler, C. Foster, et al.: Unconventional medicine in the United States: prevalence, costs, and patterns of use. *N Engl J Med.* 328:246-252 1993

103. P. Brevoort: The United States botanical market: an overview. *Herbal Gram.* 36:49-57 1996

104. Committee on the Use of Complementary and Alternative Medicine by the American Public, Board on Health Promotion and Disease Prevention, Institute of Medicine of the National Academies: Complementary and alternative medicine in the United States. 2005 National Academies Press Washington, DC

105. B. Barrett, L. Marchand, J. Scheder, et al.: Bridging the gap between conventional and alternative medicine: results of a qualitative study of patients and providers. *J Fam Pract.* 49:234-239 2000

106. W.B. Jonas, C.C. Crawford: Science and spiritual healing: a critical review of spiritual healing, "energy" medicine, and intentionality. *Altern Ther Health Med.* 9 (2):56-61 2003

107. W.C. Willett: The mediterranean diet: science and practice. *Public Health Nutr.* 9 (1A):105-110 2006

108. K.Firth, K. Smith, B.R. Sakallaris, D.M. Bellanti, C. Crawford, K.C. Avant: Healing, a concept analysis. *Global adv health med: improv healthcare outcomes worldwide.* 4 (6):44-50 2015

109. M. Lam, R. Galvin, P. Curry: Effectiveness of acupuncture for nonspecific chronic low back pain: a systematic review and meta-analysis. *Spine.* 38 (24):2124-2138 2013

110. K.J. Thomas, H. MacPherson, L. Thorpe, et al.: Randomised controlled trial of a short course of traditional acupuncture compared with usual care for persistent non-specific low back pain. *BMJ (Clinical research ed.).* 333 (7569):623 2006

111. J. Pariente, P. White, R.S. Frackowiak, G. Lewith: Expectancy and belief modulate the neuronal substrates of pain treated by acupuncture. *Neuroimage.* 25 (4):1161-1167 2005

112. S.J. Colcombe, K.I. Erickson, P.E. Scalf, et al.: Aerobic exercise training increases brain volume in aging humans. *J Gerontol A Biol Sci Med Sci.* 61 (11):1166-1170 2006

113. D.C. Cherkin, D. Eisenberg, K.J. Sherman, et al.: Randomized trial comparing traditional chinese medical acupuncture, therapeutic massage, and self-care education for chronic low back pain. *Arch Intern Med.* 161 (8):1081-1088 2001

114. J. Kabat-Zinn: Mindfulness-based interventions in context: past, present, and future. *Clin Psychol Sci Proc.* 10:144-155 2003

115. J.M. Smyth, A.A. Stone, A. Hurewitz, et al.: Effects of writing about stressful experiences on symptom reduction in patients with asthma and rheumatoid arthritis. *JAMA.* 281:1304-1309 1999

116. D.Stewart, J. Weeks, S. Bent: Utilization, patient satisfaction, and cost implications of acupuncture, massage, and naturopathic medicine offered as covered health benefits: a comparison of two delivery models. *Altern Ther.* 7:66-70 2001

117. J.E. Stahl, M.L. Dossett, A.S. LaJoie, et al.: Relaxation response and resiliency training and its effect on healthcare resource utilization. *PLoS One.* 10:e0140212 2015

118. R.L. Sarnat, J. Winterstein: Clinical and cost outcomes of an integrative medicine IPA. *J Manipulative Physiol Ther.* 27:336-347 2004

119. D. Rakel, M. Mundt, T. Ewers, et al.: Value associated with mindfulness meditation and moderate exercise intervention in acute respiratory infection: the MEPARI study. *Fam Pract.* 30:390-397 2013

120. Simmons, C. Drake, R. Snyderman: Whole health in primary care: personalized health planning and patient-centered care in a clinical setting. 2014 Duke University

121. Krause, B. Schleusser, G. Herborn, R. Rau: Response to methotrexate treatment is associated with reduced mortality in patients with severe rheumatoid arthritis. *Arthritis Rheum.* 43:14-21 2000

122. Mougil, B.M. Berman: Traditional Chinese medicine: potential for clinical treatment of rheumatoid arthritis. *Expert Rev Clin Immunol.* 10:819-822 2014

123. Brosseau, V. Welch, G. Wells, et al.: Low-level laser therapy (classes I, II, and III) for treating rheumatoid arthritis. *Cochrane Database Syst Rev.* (4):CD002049 2005

124. Wang, P. de Pablo, X. Chen, et al.: Acupuncture for pain relief in patients with rheumatoid arthritis: a systematic review. *Arthritis Rheum.* 59:1249-1256 2008

125. O'Dell, T.R. Mikuls, T.H. Taylor, et al.: Therapies for active rheumatoid arthritis after methotrexate failure. *N Engl J Med.* 369:307-318 2013

126. Pincus: Assessment of long-term outcomes of rheumatoid arthritis. *Rheum Dis Clin North Am.* 21:619-654 1995

127. Merlino, J. Curtis, T. Mikuls, et al.: Vitamin D intake is inversely associated with rheumatoid arthritis: results from the Iowa Women's Health Study. *Arthritis Rheum.* 50:72-77 2004

128. Arylaeian, F. Shahram, M. Djalali, et al.: Effect of conjugated linoleic acids, vitamin E and their combinations on the clinical outcome of Iranian adults with active rheumatoid arthritis. *Int J Rheum Dis.* 12:20-28 2009

129. Kallberg, B. Ding, L. Padyukov, et al.: Smoking is a major preventable risk factor for rheumatoid arthritis: estimations of risks after various exposures to cigarette smoke. *Ann Rheum Dis.* 70:508-511 2011

130. Linos, V.G. Kaklamani, E. Kaklamani, et al.: Dietary factors in relation to rheumatoid arthritis: a role for olive oil and cooked vegetables? *Am J Clin Nutr.* 70:1077-1082 1999

131. Henderson, R.S. Panush: Diets, nutritional supplements, and nutritional therapies in rheumatic diseases. *Rheum Dis Clin North Am.* 25:937-968 1999

132. Kojima, T. Kojima, S. Suzuki, et al.: Depression, inflammation, and pain in patients with rheumatoid arthritis. *Arthritis Rheum.* 61:1018-1024 2009

133. Zautra, M. Davis, J. Reich, et al.: Comparison of cognitive behavioral and mindfulness meditation interventions on adaptation to rheumatoid arthritis for patients with and without history of recurrent depression. *J Consult Clin Psychol.* 76:408-421 2008

134. Pradhan, M. Baumgarten, P. Langenberg, et al.: Effect of mindfulness-based stress reduction in rheumatoid arthritis patients. *Arthritis Rheum.* 57:1134-1142 2007

135. Kabat-Zinn, W. Wheeler, T. Light, et al.: Influence of a mindfulness meditation-based stress reduction intervention on rates of skin clearing in patients with moderate to severe psoriasis undergoing phototherapy (UVB) and photochemotherapy. *Psychosom Med.* 60:625-632 1998

136. Sharma: Yoga as an alternative and complementary approach for arthritis: a systematic review. *J Evid Based Complement Altern Med.* 19:51-58 2014

137. Knittle, S. Maes, V. De Gught: Psychological interventions for rheumatoid arthritis: examining the role of self-regulation with a systemic review and meta-analysis of randomized controlled trials. *Arthritis Care Res.* 62:1460-1472 2010

138. Aletaha, T. Neogi, A.J. Silman, et al.: 2010 Rheumatoid arthritis classification criteria: an American College of Rheumatology/European League against Rheumatism collaborative initiative. *Arthritis Rheum.* 62:2569-2581 2010

139. Peters, D. Symmons, D. McCarey, et al.: EULAR evidence-based recommendations for cardiovascular risk management in patients with rheumatoid arthritis and other forms of inflammatory arthritis. *Ann Rheum Dis.* 69:325-333 2010

140. Parker, K. Smarr, E. Angelone, et al.: Psychological factors, immunologic activation, and disease activity in rheumatoid arthritis. *Arthritis Care Res.* 5:196-201 1992

141. Escalante, I. Del Rincon: How much disability in rheumatoid arthritis is explained by rheumatoid arthritis?. *Arthritis Rheum.* 42:1712-1721 1999

142. Huyser, J. Parker: Stress and rheumatoid arthritis: an integrated review. *Arthritis Care Res.* 11:135-145 1998

143. Mikuls, J. Cerhan, L. Criswell, et al.: Coffee, tea, and caffeine consumption and risk of rheumatoid arthritis: results from the Iowa Women's Health Study. *Arthritis Rheum.* 46:83-91 2002

144. Heliovaara, K. Aho, P. Knekt, et al.: Coffee consumption, rheumatoid factor, and the risk of rheumatoid arthritis. *Ann Rheum Dis.* 59:631-635 2000

145. Everdingen, J. Jacobs, D. van Reesema, J. Bijlsma: Low-dose prednisone therapy for patients with early active rheumatoid arthritis: clinical efficacy, disease-modifying properties, and side effects. *Ann Intern Med.* 136:1-12 2002

146. Kirwan, Arthritis, Council Rheumatism: Low-Dose Glucocorticoid Study Group: The effect of glucocorticoids on joint destruction in rheumatoid arthritis. *N Engl J Med.* 333:142-146 1995

147. Straub, M. Cutolo: Involvement of the hypothalamic-pituitary-adrenal/gonadal axis and the peripheral nervous system in rheumatoid arthritis. *Arthritis Rheum.* 44:493-507 2001

148. Deodhar, R. Sethi, R.C. Srimal: Preliminary studies on antirheumatic activity of curcumin (deferaloyl methane). *Indian J Med Res.* 71:632-634 1980

149. Sirivastava, T. Mustafa: Ginger (Zingiber officinale) and rheumatic disorders. *Med Hypotheses.* 29:25-28 1989

150. Proudman, M.J. James, L.D. Spargo, et al.: Fish oil in recent onset rheumatoid arthritis: a randomised, double-blind controlled trial within algorithm-based drug use. *Ann Rheum Dis.* 74:89-95 2015

151. Ernst, S. Chrubasik: Phyto-anti-inflammatories: a systemic review of randomized, placebo-controlled, double-blind trials. *Rheum Dis Clin North Am.* 26:13-27 2000

152. Mangge, J. Herman, K. Schauenstein: Diet and rheumatoid arthritis: a review. *Scand J Rheumatol.* 28:201-209 1999

153. Stockl, L. Cypren, E. Chang: Gastrointestinal bleeding rates among managed care patients newly started on COX-2 inhibitors or nonselective NSAIDs. *J Manag Care Pharm.* 11:550-558 2005

154. Genovese, J. Becker, M. Schiff, et al.: Abatacept for rheumatoid arthritis refractory to tumor necrosis factor alpha inhibition. *N Engl J Med.* 353:1114-1123 2005

155. Edwards, L. Szczepanski, J. Szechinski, et al.: Efficacy of B-cell–targeted therapy with rituximab in patients with rheumatoid arthritis. *N Engl J Med.* 350:2572-2581 2004

156. Kaur, S. Kalra, S. Kaushal: Systematic review of tofacitinib: a new drug for the management of rheumatoid arthritis. *Clin Ther.* 36:1074-1086 2014

157. Bombardier, G.S. Hazelwood, P. Akhavan, et al.: Canadian Rheumatology Association recommendations for the pharmacologic management of rheumatoid arthritis with traditional and biologic disease-modifying antirheumatic drugs: Part II safety. *J Rheumatol.* 39:1583-1602 2012

158. Singh, D.E. Furst, A. Bharat, et al.: 2012 update of the 2008 American College of Rheumatology recommendations for the use of disease-modifying antirheumatic drugs and biologic agents in the treatment of rheumatoid arthritis. *Arthritis Care Res.* 64:625-639 2012

159. Choy, G. Panayi: Cytokine pathways and inflammation in rheumatoid arthritis. *N Engl J Med.* 344:907-916 2001

160. McInnes, G. Schett: The pathogenesis of rheumatoid arthritis. *N Engl J Med.* 365:2205-2219 2011

161. Arora, M. Kumar: Food allergies—leads from Ayurveda. *Indian J Med Sci.* 57 (2):57-63 2003

162. Panchal, L.C. Ward, L. Brown: Food as medicine. *Can J Physiol Pharmacol.* 91 (6):v-vi 2013

163. Klein, H. Kiat: Detox diets for toxin elimination and weight management: a critical review of the evidence. *J Hum Nutr Diet.* 28 (6):675-686 2015

164. Moore: "But we're not hypochondriacs": the changing shape of gluten-free dieting and the contested illness experience. *Soc Sci Med.* 105:76-83 2014

165. Arranz, M.A. Canela, M. Rafecas: Dietary aspects in fibromyalgia patients: results of a survey on food awareness, allergies, and nutritional supplementation. *Rheumatol Int.* 32 (9):2615-2621 2012

166. HRQoL questionnaire evaluation in lactose intolerant patients with adverse reactions to foods. *Intern Emerg Med.* 8 (6):493-496 2013

167. Volta, M.T. Bardella, A. Calabro, R. Troncone, G.R. Corazza: An Italian prospective multicenter survey on patients suspected of having non-celiac gluten sensitivity. *BMC Med.* 12:85 2014

168. Yeoh, J.P. Burton, P. Suppiah, G. Reid, S. Stebbings: The role of the microbiome in rheumatic diseases. *Curr Rheumatol Rep.* 15 (3):314 2013

169. Bjarnason, A. MacPherson, D. Hollander: Intestinal permeability: an overview. *Gastroenterology.* 108 (5):1566-1581 1995

170. Wald, D. Rakel: Behavioral and complementary approaches for the treatment of irritable bowel syndrome. *Nutr Clin Pract.* 23 (3):284-292 2008

171. Hollander: Intestinal permeability, leaky gut, and intestinal disorders. *Curr Gastroenterol Rep.* 1 (5):410-416 1999

172. Lerner, T. Matthias: Changes in intestinal tight junction permeability associated with industrial food additives explain the rising incidence of autoimmune disease. *Autoimmun Rev.* 14:479-489 2015

173. Current Concepts in Nutrition: The science and art of the elimination diet. *Altern Complement Ther.* 18 (5):251-258 2012

174. Johnson: The elimination diet and diagnosing food hypersensitivities. D. Rakel *Integrative medicine.* 2003 Saunders Philadelphia 655-659

175. Pastorello, L. Stocchi, V. Pravettoni, et al.: Role of the elimination diet in adults with food allergy. *J Allergy Clin Immunol.* 84 (4 Pt 1):475-483 1989

176. Li, R. Micheletti: Role of diet in rheumatic disease. *Rheum Dis Clin North Am.* 137:119-133 2011

177. Kanarek: Artificial food dyes and attention deficit hyperactivity disorder. *Nutr Rev.* 69 (7):385-391 2011

178. Finch, M.N. Munhutu, D.L. Whitaker-Worth: Atopic dermatitis and nutrition. *Clin Dermatol.* 28:605-614 2010 United States: 2010.

179. Vellisca, J.I. Latorre: Monosodium glutamate and aspartame in perceived pain in fibromyalgia. *Rheumatol Int.* 34 (7):1011-1013 2014

180. O'Connor Á: An overview of the role of diet in the treatment of rheumatoid arthritis. *Nutr Bull.* 39 (1):74-88 2014

181. Hagen, M.G. Byfuglien, L. Falzon, S.U. Olsen, G. Smedslund: Dietary interventions for rheumatoid arthritis. *Cochrane Database Syst Rev.* (1):CD006400 2009

182. Rountree: Roundoc rx: rheumatoid arthritis—a functional medicine approach. *Altern Complement Ther.* 20 (3):114-122 2014

183. Buchanan, S.J. Preston, P.M. Brooks, W.W. Buchanan: Is diet important in rheumatoid arthritis?. *Br J Rheumatol.* 30 (2):125-134 1991

184. Darlington: Dietary therapy for arthritis. *Rheum Dis Clin North Am.* 17 (2):273-285 1991

185. Tighe, J.R. Cummings, N.A. Afzal: Nutrition and inflammatory bowel disease: primary or adjuvant therapy. *Curr Opin Clin Nutr Metab Care.* 14:491-496 2011

186. Hobday, S. Thomas, A. O'Donovan, M. Murphy, A.J. Pinching: Dietary intervention in chronic fatigue syndrome. *J Hum Nutr Diet.* 21:141-149 2008

187. RHdeRoest, B.R. Dobbs, B.A. Chapman, et al.: The low FODMAP diet improves gastrointestinal symptoms in patients with irritable bowel syndrome: a prospective study. *Int J Clin Pract.* 67 (9):895-903 2013

188. Mooney, I. Aziz, D.S. Sanders: Non-celiac gluten sensitivity: clinical relevance and recommendations for future research. *Neurogastroenterol Motil.* 25 (11):864-871 2013

189. Boettcher, S.E. Crowe: Dietary proteins and functional gastrointestinal disorders. *Am J Gastroenterol.* 108:728-736 2013

190. Cavicchia, S.E. Steck, T.G. Hurley, et al.: A new dietary inflammatory index predicts interval changes in serum high-sensitivity C-reactive protein. *J Nutr.* 139:2365-2372 2009

191. Augustine: Integrative approach to nutrition. B. Kligler R. Lee *Integrative medicine: principles for practice.* 2004 McGraw Hill New York

192. Pattison, D.P. Symmons, M. Lunt, et al.: Dietary beta-cryptoxanthin and inflammatory polyarthritis: results from a population-based prospective study. *Am J Clin Nutr.* 82:451-455 2005

193. Casas, E. Sacanella, R. Estruch: The immune protective effect of the Mediterranean diet against chronic low-grade inflammatory diseases. *Endocr Metab Immune Disord Drug Targets.* 14:245-254 2014

194. West, H. Renz, M.C. Jenmalm, et al.: The gut microbiota and inflammatory no communicable diseases: associations and potentials for gut microbiota therapies. *J Allergy Clin Immunol.* 135:3-13 2015

195. Jones, J. Versalovic: Probiotic Lactobacillus reuteri biofilms produce antimicrobial and anti-inflammatory factors. *BMC Microbiol.* 9:35 2009

196. Sun, E.B. Chang: Exploring gut microbes in human health and disease: pushing the envelope. *Genes Dis.* 1:132-139 2014

197. Willcox, B.J. Willcox, H. Todoriki, et al.: The Okinawan diet: health implications of a low-calorie, nutrient-dense, antioxidant-rich dietary pattern low in glycemic load. *J Am Coll Nutr.* 28 (Suppl):500S-516S 2009

198. Grey, M. Bolland: Clinical trial evidence and use of fish oil supplements. *JAMA Intern Med.* 174:460-462

199. Fernando, I.J. Martins, K.G. Goozee, et al.: The role of dietary coconut for the prevention and treatment of Alzheimer's disease: potential mechanisms of action. *Br J Nutr.* 114:1-14 2015

200. Vitaglione, I. Mennella, R. Ferracane, et al.: Whole-grain wheat consumption reduces inflammation in a randomized controlled trial on overweight and obese subjects with unhealthy dietary and lifestyle behaviors: role of polyphenols bound to cereal. *Am J Clin Nutr.* 101:251-261 2015

201. Herder, M. Peltonen, W. Koenig, et al.: Anti-inflammatory effect of lifestyle changes in the Finnish Diabetes Prevention Study. *Diabetologia.* 52:433-442 2009

202. Martinez, J.M. Lattimer, K.L. Hubach, et al.: Gut microbiome composition is linked to whole grain-induced immunological improvements. *ISME J.* 7:269-280 2013

203. Nanri, D. Yoshida, T. Yamaji, et al.: Dietary patterns and C-reactive protein in Japanese men and women. *Am J Clin Nutr.* 87:1488-1496 2008

204. Hermsdorff, Abete I. Zulet MÁ, et al.: A legume-based hypocaloric diet reduces proinflammatory status and improves metabolic features in overweight/obese subjects. *Eur J Nutr.* 50:61-69 2011

205. Ley, Q. Sun, W.C. Willett, et al.: Associations between red meat intake and biomarkers of inflammation and glucose metabolism in women. *Am J Clin Nutr.* 99:352-360 2014

206. Montonen, H. Boeing, A. Fritsche, et al.: Consumption of red meat and whole-grain bread in relation to biomarkers of obesity, inflammation, glucose metabolism and oxidative stress. *Eur J Nutr.* 52:337-345 2013

207. Larsson, N. Orsini: Red meat and processed meat consumption and all-cause mortality: a meta-analysis. *Am J Epidemiol.* 179:282-289 2014

208. Li, A. Ng, N.J. Mann, et al.: Contribution of meat fat to dietary arachidonic acid. *Lipids.* 33:437-440 1998

209. Zheng, S.A. Lee: Well-done meat intake, heterocyclic amine exposure, and cancer risk. *Nutr Cancer.* 61:437-446 2009

210. P. Couture, C. Richard, et al.: Impact of dairy products on biomarkers of inflammation: a systematic review of randomized controlled nutritional intervention studies. *Am J Clin Nutr.* 97:706-717 2013

211. Mozaffarian, E.B. Rimm: Fish intake, contaminants, and human health: evaluating the risks and the benefits. *JAMA.* 296:1885-1899 2006

212. Ganjali, A. Sahebkar, E. Mahdipour, et al.: Investigation of the effects of curcumin on serum cytokines in obese individuals: a randomized controlled trial. *Scientific World J.* 2014:898361 2014

213. Akazawa, Y. Choi, A. Miyaki, et al.: Curcumin ingestion and exercise training improve vascular endothelial function in postmenopausal women. *Nutr Res.* 32:795-799 2012

214. Kuptniratsaikul, P. Dajpratham, W. Taechaarpornkul, et al.: Efficacy and safety of Curcuma domestica extracts compared with ibuprofen in patients with knee osteoarthritis: a multicenter study. *Clin Interv Aging.* 9:451-458 2014

215. Hanai, T. Iida, K. Takeuchi, et al.: Curcumin maintenance therapy for ulcerative colitis: randomized, multicenter, double-blind, placebo-controlled trial. *Clin Gastroenterol Hepatol.* 4:1502-1506 2006

216. Mueller, S. Hobiger, A. Jungbauer: Anti-inflammatory activity of extracts from fruits, herbs and spices. *Food Chem.* 122:987-996 2010

217. Allgrove, G. Davison: Dark chocolate/cocoa polyphenols and oxidative stress. *Polyphenols in human health and disease.* 2014 Elsevier Inc. 241-251

218. Stote, B.A. Clevidence, J.A. Novotny, et al.: Effect of cocoa and green tea on biomarkers of glucose regulation, oxidative stress, inflammation and hemostasis in obese adults at risk for insulin resistance. *Eur J Clin Nutr.* 66:1153-1159 2012

219. West, M.D. McIntyre, M.J. Piotrowski, et al.: Effects of dark chocolate and cocoa consumption on endothelial function and arterial stiffness in overweight adults. *Br J Nutr.* 111:653-661 2014

220. Papanikolaou, J. Brooks, C. Reider, et al.: U.S. adults are not meeting recommended levels for fish and omega-3 fatty acid intake: results of an analysis using observational data from NHANES 2003-2008. *Nutr J.* 13:31 2014

221. Vaghef-Mehrabany, B. Alipour, A. Homayouni-Rad, et al.: Probiotic supplementation improves inflammatory status in patients with rheumatoid arthritis. *Nutrition.* 30:430-435 2014

222. Pennebaker: Opening up: the healing power of expressing emotions. 1997 Guilford Press New York

223. Klein, A. Boals: Expressive writing can increase working memory capacity. *J Exp Psychol Gen.* 130:520-533 2001

224. Pennebaker: Expressive writing in a clinical setting: a brief practical guide to expressive writing for therapists and counselors. *Indep Pract.* 30:23-25 2010

225. Halpert, D. Rybin, G. Doros: Expressive writing is a promising therapeutic modality for the management of IBS: a pilot study. *Am J Gastroenterol.* 105:2440-2448 2010

226. Banburey: Wounds heal more quickly if patients are relieved of stress: a review of research by susanne scott and colleagues from king's college. London. presented at the annual conference of the british psychological society *BMJ.* 327:522 2003

227. Cameron, G. Nicholls: Expression of stressful experiences through writing: effects of a self-regulation manipulation for pessimists and optimists. *Health Psychol.* 17:84-92 1998

228. Fortney, M. Taylor: Meditation in medical practice: a review of the evidence and practice. *Prim Care.* 37:81-90 2010

229. Helms: The basic, clinical, and speculative science of acupuncture. *Acupuncture energetics: a clinical approach for physicians.* 1995 Medical Acupuncture Publishers Berkeley, CA 19-69

230. Edzard, A.R. White: Prospective studies of the safety of acupuncture: a systematic review. *Am J Med.* 110:481-485 2001

231. MacPherson, K. Thomas, S. Walters, M. Fitter: The York Acupuncture Safety Study: prospective survey of 34,000 treatments by traditional acupuncturists. *BMJ.* 323:486-487 2001

232. Melchart, W. Weidenhammer, A. Streng: Prospective investigation of adverse effects of acupuncture in 97,733 patients. *Arch Intern Med.* 164:104-105 2004

233. Ambrosio, K. Bloor, H. MacPherson: Costs and consequences of acupuncture as a treatment for chronic pain: a systematic review of economic evaluations conducted alongside randomised controlled trials. *Complement Ther Med.* 20:364-374 2012

234. Kim, H. Lee, Y. Chae, H.J. Park, H. Lee: A systematic review of cost-effectiveness analyses alongside randomised controlled trials of acupuncture. *Acupunct Med.* 30:273-285 2012

235. Medscape. https://www.medscape.com

ABOUT THE AUTHOR

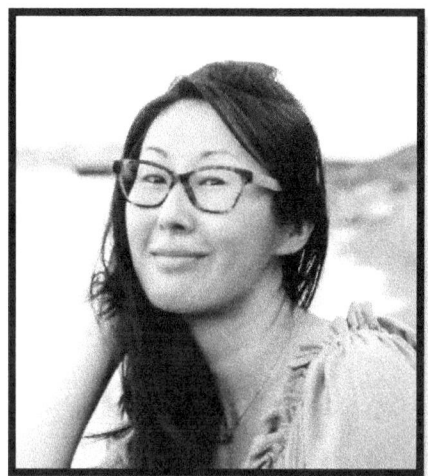

Donica Liu Baker, MD, FACR is a rheumatologist practicing the art of medicine in her beloved hometown of St. Louis, Missouri. As a Kinesiology major in college at the University of Michigan-Ann Arbor, she developed an early passion for helping patients improve their mobility, which evolved into an interest in arthritis and autoimmune diseases.

She completed most of her medical education, including rheumatology fellowship, at the University of Missouri in Columbia. For her, the best part of being in medicine is having a window of perspective to understand humanity from all walks of life, and getting to see points of view that are different from her own.

She enjoys spending time with her family and friends, writing, and hiking with her dogs Sasha and Coco. She also dabbles in yoga, meditation, practicing piano, singing at her church, and exploring activities around St. Louis city.

Visit www.donicabaker.com.

ALSO WRITTEN BY THE AUTHOR

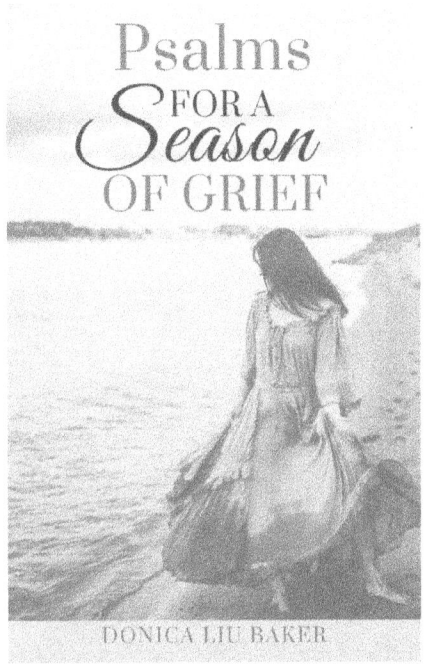

Psalms for a Season of Grief

Grief is a universal experience, but so rarely talked about or expressed. After a prolonged hospitalization and the loss of her young son to a devastating illness, the author experienced a journey of grief and mourning that left her broken, but also gave her a spiritual awakening and a renewed sense of purpose towards life. In her book, she shares the verses from the book of Psalms that shaped her transformation, and offers hope and encouragement for others who are experiencing grief and loss in any form. Available to order on Amazon.com.

ALSO WRITTEN BY THE AUTHOR

The Psoriatic Arthritis Roadmap

Navigating an Integrative Approach

Dr. Donica Baker

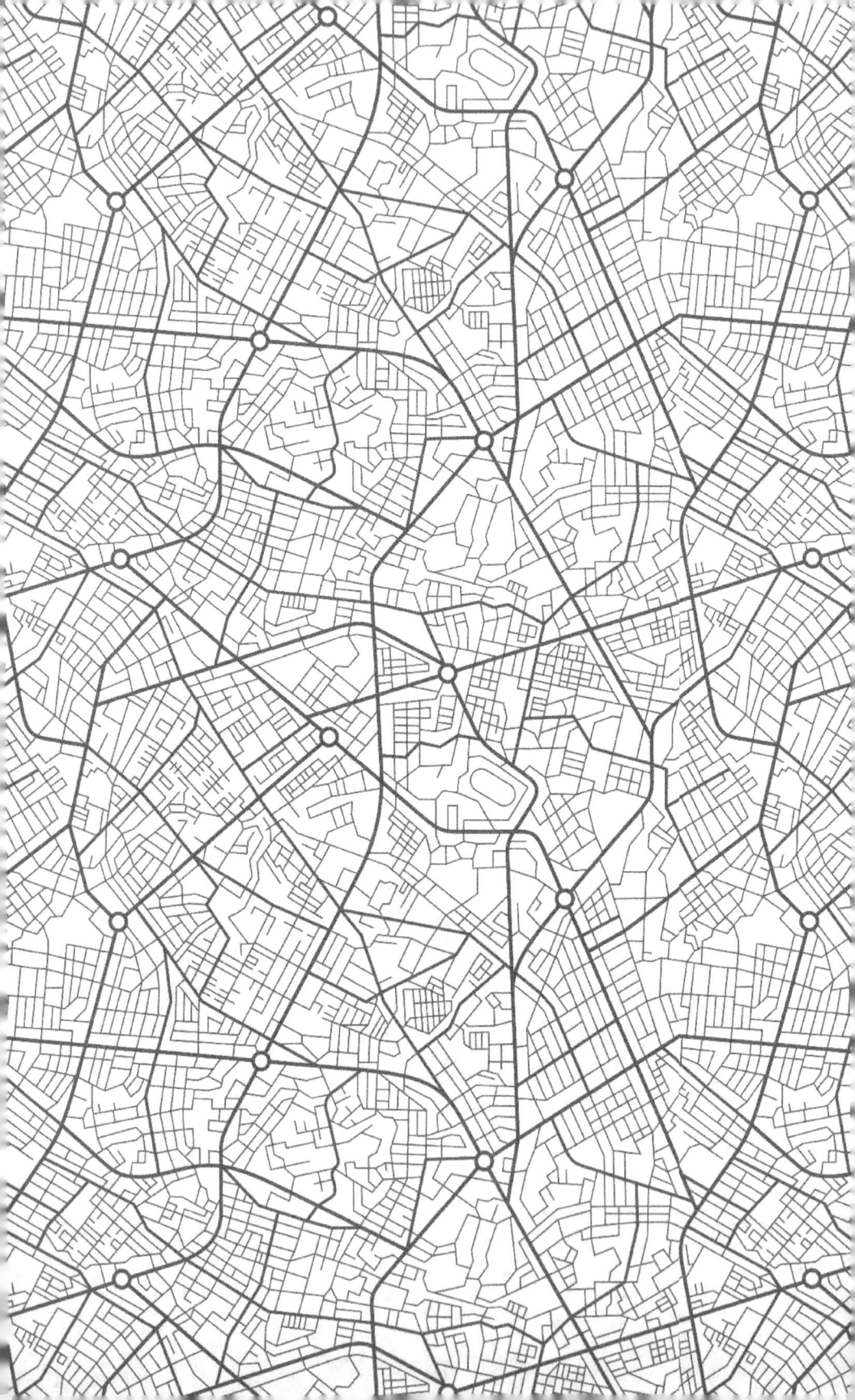

www.ingramcontent.com/pod-product-compliance
Lightning Source LLC
Chambersburg PA
CBHW052309220526
45472CB00001B/44